TRANSPLANT
... LIFE'S SECOND CHANCE

MARGOT MAURICE

TRANSPLANT... LIFE'S SECOND CHANCE
Copyright (c) Margot Maurice 2017

ISBN-13: 978-1544832937

ISBN-10: 1544832931

All rights reserved. No part of this book may be reproduced in any form or by any electronic or mechanical means including information storage and retrieval systems, without permission in writing from the author. The only exception is by a reviewer, who may quote short excerpts in a review.

AN INTRODUCTION...

A New Start at Life

Organ transplants are becoming more common place these days than they were even twenty years ago. When I was diagnosed with cardiomyopathy in 1984 I was considered not a suitable candidate for transplant as the age range accepted then was forty years and younger.

I was in my fifty second year.

Since I started writing about the transplant subject, I have been able to see the differences in people's stories and in the way they have handled this life changing surgery.

One thing I have noticed is that an essential element for everyone is to have a supportive partner and/or family. It's not just the physical aspects, but most certainly in the build up, there is a lot of emphasis on the psychological aspects the patient will be facing during the rehabilitation period.

I would at this stage like to sincerely thank the people who have been most helpful in giving me their stories. This has been a brave decision as it often opens up old memories and makes the recipient face that period of time, when they felt absolutely frightened of what was to come. Trying hard to switch their thinking into how much better they would feel when it was all over is difficult, yet it is a huge decision to make, not only to decide to have the surgery, but then to relive it all when recalling their own story.

We all like to think we are strong and can face anything that is put before us, but unfortunately our mind plays tricks quite often and pushes us into taking part in all those 'what ifs.'

What if it doesn't work for me?

What if I become a different person when I have the heart of someone else?

And then the big one... what if I don't survive?

Our mind takes a battering during these periods of doubt. We try desperately to stay positive, but many of us have heard those stories of how some people take on characteristics of the donor whose heart is now housed in a different body... not the donor's.

I asked this question of several transplant patients but none seemed to have a definitive answer, so I came to the conclusion it depends on how much leeway we give our imagination and how many of the patients want to be a different person. Religious, spiritual and psychological beliefs come into this conundrum, so there is no hard and fast answer..

Scientists will dismiss this idea, as will some folk whose religious beliefs do not allow them to think about such things. Free thinkers might give it some consideration, but the majority of people will come back to the thought, "What does it matter? It is my heart now and part of my physical body."

As I am a strong believer in mind/body medicine, I tend to think that the brain/mind will influence the new heart to be the body's new pump with a job to do.

There is no wrong or right answer to this complex question and as you will read, each patient who receives a new heart, has a different story to tell in some way, as all of us come into this life with a different set of beliefs... some inherited, some learned and some acquired from peers and opinions change as we mature.

CHAPTER 1

History

One of the first mentions about the possibility of a heart transplantation was by American medical researcher Simon Fleecer. He declared in a reading of his paper on "Tendencies in Pathology" in the University of Chicago in 1907, that it would be possible in the future for diseased human organ substitution. He suggested surgery, including arteries, stomach, kidneys and heart will be common place

In 1945 the Soviet Pathologist Nikolai Sinitsyn successfully transplanted a heart from one frog to another frog, and from one dog to another dog. Both recipients survived the procedure.

On January 23, 1964, Dr. James Hardy performed the first heart transplant at the University of Mississippi Medical Center in Jackson, MS, in which the heart of a chimpanzee was transplanted into the chest of Boyd Rush (age 68). This was decided as a last effort trying to save the dying man as no human heart was available. Rush died after 90 minutes.

Hardy dealt with severe criticism for performing the transplant, but the operation manifested the possibility of human heart transplantation. Three years later, the first successful human-to-human heart transplantation was performed in 1967 by a South African cardiac surgeon, Christiaan Barnard.

Although Norman Shumway is widely regarded as the father of transplantation, the world's first adult human heart transplant was performed by the aforementioned Barnard the South African cardiac surgeon, utilizing the techniques developed and perfected by Shumway and Richard Lower.

Barnard performed the first transplant on Louis Washkansky on December 3, 1967 at the Groote Schuur Hospital in Cape Town, South Africa.

Adrian Kamtrowitz performed the world's first pediatric heart transplant on December 6, 1967, at Maimonidea Hospital in Brooklyn New York, barely three days after Christiaan Barnard's pioneering procedure.

Norman Shumway performed the first adult heart transplant in the United States on January 6, 1968, at the Stanford University Hospital.

Worldwide, about 3,500 heart transplants are performed annually. The vast majority of these are performed in the United States (2,000-2,300 annually). Cedars-Sinai Medical Center in Los Angeles, California, currently is the largest heart transplant center in the world, having performed 119 adult transplants in 2013 alone. About 800,000 people have NYHA Class 1V- heart failure symptoms, indicating advanced heart failure. The great disparity between the number of patients needing transplants and the number of procedures being performed spurred research into the transplantation of non-human hearts into humans after 1993. Xenografts from other species and man-made artificial hearts are two less successful alternatives to allografts. (*a tissue graft from a donor of the same species as the recipient but not genetically identical.*)

However, in the Southern Hemisphere heart transplants are recorded in Australia. And according to information from the Heart Foundation Australia, heart transplants since the first successful one in 1984 performed by the late Doctor Victor Chang AC, at St Vincent's Hospital Sydney have increased in numbers with locations now in Sydney, Melbourne, Brisbane and Perth.

As a gifted surgeon, a respected humanitarian and skilled campaigner, Dr Victor Chang was a pioneer of the modern era of heart transplantation. His achievements include developing Australia's National Heart Transplant Program at St Vincent's hospital, which has since performed more than 1200 successful heart, as well as heart-lung, and single lung transplants since 1984. He also saw the incredible value of research – playing a key role in development of an artificial heart valve and, in later years, an artificial heart.

Victor Chang (Yam Him) was born in Shanghai of Australian-born Chinese parents. He came to Australia in 1953 to complete his secondary schooling at Christian Brothers College. He graduated from Sydney University with a Bachelor of Medicine, Bachelor of Surgery in 1962.

In 1966 Victor Chang became a Fellow of the Royal College of Surgeons at the age of 30. Initially he trained in general surgery in England, but he commenced serious training in cardiac and thoracic surgery at the Brampton Hospital for Chest Diseases in London.

It was in London that he met and married his wife, Ann. After two years at the Mayo Clinic in the US, where he was chief resident, he returned to Sydney in 1972 to join the elite St Vincent's cardio-thoracic team. This included Dr Harry Windsor and Dr Mark Shanahan. In 1973 he was made a Fellow of the Australasian College of Surgeons and in 1975 he became a Fellow of the American College of Surgeons.

A pioneer of the modern era of heart transplantation, Victor Chang was responsible for the establishment of the National Heart Transplant Unit at St Vincent's Hospital in 1984, lobbying politicians and raising funds for its ongoing work.

In 1986, he was appointed a Companion of the Order of Australia for his 'service to international relations between Australia and China and to medical science'.

In 1991, Chang died tragically after being shot in a failed extortion attempt against him. His legacy includes, the creation of the Victor Chang Cardiac Research Institute, being voted Australian of the Century at the People's Choice Awards, and the establishment of the Victor Chang, Lowy Packer Building in St Vincent's Hospital.

References. https://en.wikipedia.org/
http://www.victorchang.edu.au/home/about/victor-chang

CHAPTER 2

After the event

After an organ transplant, most patients feel comparatively better, although their recovery rates vary case by case. They go on to enjoy a significantly improved quality of life, although this tends to happen also case by case, as far as time spans go.

One recipient commented on how it felt to be no longer on a fluid restriction. All heart failure patients are on limited amounts of fluids for quite a long time prior to their surgery, so this patient was overjoyed to have this early change.

But they are also likely to face big health challenges, in some cases.

The recovery rate varies with the age of the recipient, how long they have been unwell and how long they have been waiting for the donor organ. They are all well prepared by the medical team working with them on what to expect.

You will read more of these situations in the following patient's stories.

The first patient story is Gaylynn who lives in Melbourne, Victoria

in Australia with her ever attentive husband. He has been there for her, right from the start and this has had a huge bearing on Gaylynn's ability to come through the ups and downs of the experience. She has also been able to maintain a positive outlook through it all and that has been a huge help in her recovery.

Gaylynn's Story:

"Trying to think back to when there was something that stood out as seeming 'not quite right', I remember thinking that, although I attended aerobic classes and was therefore reasonably fit, when I pruned the roses and then bent over to collect up the prunings I had a 'strange feeling.'

Apart from that anything else was thought to be stress associated with work.

One day about a month after my 50th birthday, when I was at work I felt so bad, that I made an appointment to see a city doctor. The earliest appointment was just after lunch and I somehow managed to still join friends for lunch. The doctor finally suggested, that he try out his new portable ECG machine. I could soon see by his face that something wasn't quite right and he quickly called another doctor. An ambulance was organized to take me to Epworth Hospital in Richmond, an inner Melbourne suburb. My husband Ross was contacted at work and he jumped on a tram, arriving just as I was loaded into the ambulance. He came along for the ride, so I was lucky to have him with me when I was taken into Emergency. This was just the first of a number of times that he was able to be with me for support in emergency situations. I know I have been so lucky in this regard. I had more important things on my mind while in Emergency, although I wanted to go back to work to tidy my desk!

I was immediately diagnosed with Ventricular Tachycardia (VT). After two attempts at ablation, the second only a couple of weeks later because the leading world expert (a Canadian) happened to be visiting Melbourne to demonstrate the latest equipment. It was confirmed that ablation was not possible, due to my heart kicking off from within a muscle. Medication was prescribed.

Cardiac Ablation is a procedure to disable a small amount of heart tissue in very specific places. The heart has many electrical connections. Sometimes these connections can become abnormal and can cause the heart to beat very fast and irregularly. By disabling some of the problem areas, the heart rhythm can be improved or made normal. Ablation is done for people who:

- *Have Wolf-Parkinson-White syndrome.*
- *Have other fast heart rhythms known as tachycardia.*
- *Have tried medications for an abnormal heart rhythm that resulted in:*
- *No success.*
- *Side effects.*
- *May have a high risk heart beat (arrhythmia that could result in death.)*

Although medically I should have been able to return to work in a couple of weeks it took much longer and looking back, this might have been due to anxiety.

Three years went by and I continued in my busy job. Quite a lot of the time I would find it difficult to walk the couple of blocks to work from the tram stop and I knew I just wasn't feeling right.

On our Labor Day Long Weekend in March 2000 I felt totally 'strange'. I couldn't sit down, lie down, had some trouble breathing and generally felt awful. We returned from the country late at night and I went to Epworth Hospital the following morning. It was then discovered that the condition of my heart had deteriorated. As the cardiologist walked out the door on his way to the USA for a Conference he told me I was a very sick lady. Luckily we have many world-class cardiologists here in Melbourne.

Transplant...Life's Second Chance

From that day in March 2000 my life has been one of 'real adventure'. I was transferred from Epworth Hospital to Melbourne Private Hospital for surgery at Royal Melbourne Hospital. We were then told that my best option was to be sent to Westmead Hospital in Sydney, where Professor David Ross was the leader in the field.

I clearly remember the trip to Sydney.

It was a clear crisp morning when I was taken by ambulance to Essendon Airport and transferred to the Air Ambulance. I actually felt fine and found it strange not to be allowed to sit up and enjoy the perfect flight. It was a similar day when I arrived at Bankstown Airport. Just as well, I was on the stretcher on the tarmac waiting for the ambulance to take me to Westmead Hospital. The air ambulance officers were getting anxious, as they were to collect a patient from Wangaratta on the way back to Melbourne.

I can't remember much after my arrival at Westmead Hospital. Apparently I had been heavily sedated for about seven days following the open heart surgery which was touch and go and took about 10 hours. There was no definitive diagnosis and so it was called, giant cell cardiomyopathy. The cause is still a mystery.

As I opened my eyes, I saw my elderly parents walking in the door in ICU and all I could think of was 'I have to make it'. I couldn't speak because of the length of time I had the tube in my throat and so on an alphabet board (difficult without my glasses) my first question was "Where am I?" Ross had to make a quick trip back to Melbourne and my parents telephoned to let him know that he would see a great improvement on his return. Luckily this was the time of the unbelievable discounted air fares.

Apparently while I was in ICU family and friends had been visiting and had been massaging my feet, which was very important. One friend reminds me of how I used to wave – just like the Queen! The nurse assigned to me in ICU was very stern and would take no nonsense from me. She put on her gumboots and it was off to the shower, no matter how awful you felt. Probably did me a favor. The medical staff said I was a very strong person. I didn't feel that way. I am not a religious person but many people prayed for me and I was given a dab of Lourdes water by a friend before the surgery.

It was hoped that I wouldn't need a defibrillator but unfortunately my VT still needed to be controlled. So a bit more surgery.

After seven weeks in hospital the first thing I noticed when I went outside was the sound of the birds. It was lovely. Ross had been able to have time off work and stayed in a hostel in the hospital grounds – handy for visiting and doing the washing!

We flew back to Melbourne.

Some people have a defibrillator which rarely or never goes off. Unfortunately mine went off the morning after arriving home. I had just showered. The fear of this happening became associated with having a shower. We live close to a major hospital, the Austin and Repatriation Medical Center, where I was able to have my defibrillator interrogated which was comforting. During the next few weeks I visited my cardiologist where adjustments to the defibrillator setting and medication were needed.

I was in and out of hospital due to defibrillator episodes (about six months apart) which required calling an ambulance. I was lucky on all occasions that Ross was able to be with me in Emergency. On the first occasion Ross and a couple of neighbors were with me, on the second occasion a neighbor called my cardiologist and by coincidence Ross had gone there to his office at the hospital to collect a prescription and actually heard the call on the loud speaker. I called it Hotel Epworth and felt quite at home knowing so many of the staff. I was requiring more and more support. It was arranged for me to have an interview with a representative from the Alfred Hospital Heart Transplant Team. It was not until later as my condition deteriorated that I was accepted for assessment for the Transplant List.

The assessment is very thorough – from tests for TB to the health of your teeth! Interviews with you and your carer are undertaken by cardiologists, transplant coordinators, dieticians, physiotherapists, social workers to name but a few. Results are presented to a forum of all the medical personnel involved and the result is given to you by a consultant cardiologist.

As you wait on that day you wonder whether you have 'passed the test'. If they say you are unsuccessful you would be very disappointed. If the answer is yes, you are scared but you know that you are very very lucky. I was given the wonderful news in May 2002 and was told that they hoped I would receive my new heart by Christmas but of course no-one knows. I was given my pager.

We attended the Heart Lung Transplant Association Christmas BBQ and I was encouraged by meeting so many people who had had transplants – some of whom I had met in the pre-transplant information sessions just months before and others who had their transplants fourteen years back.

I am lucky to be living in Melbourne, only a 45 minute drive from the Alfred Hospital so life went on much the same for us. Others who live in Western Australia (lungs), South Australia or Tasmania (heart and lungs) have to come to Melbourne once they are on the active list. Some wait for a couple of years. How much more difficult it is for them – both financially and with support. Carers often have to give up their jobs. Families are split up for a considerable time.

On a regular pre-transplant visit I discussed a red mark that had appeared on my skin around the area of the defibrillator. The cardiologist at the Alfred Hospital consulted with my cardiologist at Epworth Hospital and it was decided that my defibrillator should be re-sited to ensure the red mark wasn't an infection. The operation would have to be at Royal Melbourne Hospital and once again I was booked into Melbourne Private Hospital.

The night before I was to be admitted I ended up in Epworth Hospital. I remember coming back from a friend's place and not feeling very well. The next thing I remember is opening my eyes and my neighbor was sitting on the bed beside me saying that the ambulance is on the way and Ross would be home soon. He was once again able to be with me in Emergency. Apparently I had pressed my Safety Link buzzer. Later I wanted to find out the details and apparently I told them my defibrillator had gone off and I needed an ambulance. The front door was open and I was on the bed – amazing!

I had just been loaded into the ambulance at Epworth to go to Melbourne Private when the ambulance drivers and I heard a beeping noise. As it wasn't anything to do with them I suddenly remembered I had the beeper in my bag. I asked them to ring the Alfred Hospital because we might be going there instead. Turned out it was a false alarm.

The repositioning operation was supposed to be fairly minor but I felt pretty bad after it. Didn't really want to go home.

Around 9.30 pm on Sunday 22 December 2003 I said to Ross that he should put on the mobile phone while he is on the internet. At 10.20 pm the mobile phone rang. It was **'the'** *call. What did I say? "Oh, I only had an operation a couple of weeks ago." The response, "Don't you want this?" And of course I answered, "Yes, I'm sorry." We arrived at the Alfred at midnight and the operation took place around 6.30 am on Monday 23 December. I remember being placed on the operating table and all the nurses were so cold they had blankets around them while they waited for the action. The procedure took about seven hours. And so it did happen before Christmas.*

I recovered exceptionally well, apart from only being able to have soup on Christmas Day while in ICU! The ward staff were amazed with my progress. I was discharged on day 11 but not before I had been on the treadmill in the gym.

All heart and lung transplant patients together with their carers make a commitment to a 12-week post-transplant program. This involves information sessions on medication, nutrition, exercise and attending the gym three times a week. This is where I noticed my diagnosis on the front cover of my gym file – near end cardiomyopathy – and I thought to myself 'just as well it didn't say very near end'! You have a biopsy and other tests weekly at first, then monthly, two monthly and at larger time intervals as time went on. The day after the biopsy you see a consultant for the results. So in the early days you are attending the Alfred Hospital four days a week. The support given by the Alfred Heart/Lung Transplant Team is exceptional.

So where am I now – 10 months since my transplant? Medically my reports couldn't be better and my medication has been reduced. I attend the local YMCA gym three times a week and tai chi once a week. I still have a bit of a problem walking some distance. I suffer with some anxiety, something which I have had on and off over the years. I was able to attend a number of sessions with a psychologist at the Alfred Hospital and this has helped considerably. But what about all the things I can do now – all the housework, socializing and we have been able to go away on holiday including a trip to Sydney to attend a wedding (and I even danced to the tune YMCA – a big achievement!)

The day after, I had spoken to a couple with whom we had to share a table at a busy restaurant. I began talking to the couple who explained that they had sold their house and were about to leave for Queensland in their motor home. They had traveled this way before and enjoyed it immensely. I commented that it is good to travel when you are healthy and that I'd had some heart problems. The wife then mentioned that she had been diagnosed with cardiomyopathy. She said I was only the second person she had met and it was so good to talk to someone who understood how she felt. I was inspired by her because it seemed to me that she was brave to do all that traveling around Australia. I mentioned the Cardiomyopathy Association. She already had the application form but because of the traveling hadn't yet joined. So I hope I get to meet her again.

Finally, it would have been impossible for me to have this second chance at life without the kindness of my donor family. I felt I was ready to write my thank you letter to the donor family at the time of my six month anniversary. Letters are sent in a sealed envelope through the Red Cross to the family and it is their choice as to whether they open it. One day I received mail which was enclosed in a sealed envelope. I had no hesitation in opening the envelope. It was a lovely letter from my donor's family.

To them, I will always be grateful. But there are so many people who have been involved in helping me – family and friends who supported me, medical staff who got me through to having the heart transplant, the friendship of Cardiomyopathy Australia members with a special mention for Bob Christelow who visited me weekly and patiently taught me how to do tapestry.

At Westmead I had been diagnosed with Giant Cell Cardiomyopathy (usually associated with Giant Cell Myocarditis) but because I wasn't aware of anyone who was suffering with Cardiomyopathy it left me with a feeling of not knowing what was going on."

Myocarditis is a complex disease because multiple pathogenetic mechanisms play a role. While these mechanisms appear to act in a chronological cascade, they undoubtedly overlap in some cases, rendering diagnosis and treatment difficult. Ultimately, dilated cardiomyopathy (DCM) may result.

Reference://http://www.differencebetween.com/difference-between-my

So how did I get to know about the Cardiomyopathy Association now referred to as Cardiomyopathy Australia?

It was only recently that I came across a copy of my initial application and noticed that I had put down that I heard about it from the hospital. But it was my husband who made the effort for both of us. I am sure it gave him an anchor with those who were going through the same experience - my life changed but so did his. My first recollection of going to a meeting was one held at Royal Melbourne Hospital - I probably needed a wheelchair. I recall immediately being made to feel welcome. From then on I had a feeling of not being alone with my illness. From that initial meeting, during the time of my transplant and ever since, I know there are people who understand and care about me. People need to be aware of the value of support groups and Cardiomyopathy Australia has contact people around Australia who can be of assistance."

CHAPTER 3

Some interesting facts

The following statistics on organ donation in Australia have been compiled from the Australian and New Zealand Organ Donor

1500 patients waiting for a transplant.
435 Organ donors.
1,241 transplant recipients.
2015 Breakdown is 703 kidney, 264 liver, 95 heart,47 pancreas, 195 lung transplants.

Notable recipients around the world

At the time of his death on August 10, 2009, Tony Huesman was the world's longest living heart transplant recipient, having survived for 30 years, 11 months and 10 days, before dying of cancer.

Huesman received a heart in 1978 at the age of 20 after viral pneumonia severely weakened his heart. The operation was performed at Stanford University.

As of December 2013, the record holder for longest living heart recipient was Englishman John McCafferty, 71. He received his heart on 20 October 1982.

Former Vice President of the United States, Dick Cheney received a heart transplant on March 24, 2012. Because he was 71 years old at the time of the surgery, it sparked discussions about the upper age of transplant patients.

John McCafferty had his heart transplant at Harefield Hospital in October 1982.

- He was told the life-saving surgery was only likely to last five years.
- Officially became world's longest surviving heart transplant patient in 2013.
- Wife, Ann, 70, said surgery allowed them to 'travel the world together.

Reference Daily Mail UK

Is age a barrier in receiving a heart transplant?

In the US it is considered that in the case of Mr Dick Cheney's it will soon be the exception and not the rule.

Transplant centers don't expect a flood of older patients anytime soon. Most 70-something adults with failing hearts aren't good candidates for these demanding surgeries, experts say, and in any event, organs are just too scarce.

Each transplant center decides on its own, which older patients to accept for transplant and under what circumstances, and policies vary across the country. Some centers, like the Cleveland Clinic and Johns Hopkins Medicine, will operate on patients in their early or even middle 70s. Other centers will not.

Just a decade ago, people 65 and older were routinely rejected for heart transplants at all but a few institutions. But in 2006, the International Society for Heart and Lung Transplantation issued new guidelines saying that heart failure patients should be considered for transplants up to age 70.

Read more: *http://www.dailymail.co.uk/health/article-3442071/Longest-surviving-heart-transplant-patient-dies-aged-73-blood-poisoning-kidney-failure-33-years-operation.html#ixzz4KSy1cVxd*

Follow us: *@MailOnline* on Twitter | *DailyMail* on Facebook

The voluntary guidelines reflected advances in transplantation and a growing older population in better health and with longer lifespans than in decades past. The society left open the possibility of transplanting hearts into patients over age 70, as long as recipients were otherwise in very good health.

"Many of these older patients can transition to an even older age while maintaining a very good quality of life. Why would we deny someone that opportunity?" said Dr. Mandeep Mehra, executive director of the Center for Advanced Heart Disease at Brigham and Women's Hospital in Boston and chairman of the committee that drew up the society's new criteria.

The new policy has led to a gradual expansion of heart transplants in older patients. But the frequency of these procedures has not risen dramatically, because of an acute shortage of donor hearts, strict eligibility standards for potential recipients and caution at transplant centers that do not want to jeopardize success averages with risky operations.

In 2006, 243 patients age 65 and older in the United States received new hearts; last year, that number was 332, according to data from the national Organ Procurement and Transplantation Network. (Data strictly on patients 70 and older is not available, according to the network.)

More than 500 people age 65 and older were waiting for new hearts. In 2011, 55 patients in this age group died before organs became available.

Heart transplantation involves major, invasive surgery and burdensome follow-up care; two dozen biopsies are usually performed on each patient in the first two years alone. So medical centers generally subject people in the 65-plus age bracket to especially rigorous evaluation before approving them as candidates.

This is a much discussed topic and there appears to be as many experts discouraging older recipients for heart transplantation as there are those having the opposite view so it would appear that there are many deciding factors such as general health, availability of a suitable heart and a surgeon who believes he can help his elderly patients.

References :www.sciencedirect.com/science/article/p

CHAPTER 4

Do Cells have memory?

There are quite a few people worldwide who believe that every cell in our body has memory thus influencing the thinking and behavior of a transplant recipient. This is a contentious issue and the reader might immediately dismiss such a theory, but it does us all some good to look at other people's views on this matter and take from it either nothing at all or something that might resonate with some who will state, "Well maybe this is possible."

I am one who believes there is no such thing as an impossibility and so I explore all options.

In 1997, a book titled *A Change of Heart* was published that described the apparent personality changes experienced by the writer, **Claire Sylvia** now deceased.

Sylvia received a heart and lung transplant at Yale-New Haven Hospital in 1988. She reported noticing that various attitudes, habits and tastes changed following her surgery. She had inexplicable cravings for foods she had previously disliked. For example, though she was a health-conscious dancer and choreographer, upon leaving the hospital she had an uncontrollable urge to go to a Kentucky Fried Chicken outlet and order chicken nuggets, a food she never previously ate.

Claire Sylvia, a former Hull, USA, resident who was the first person in New England to undergo a heart-lung transplant, died at age 69, 21 years after the operation. Her story received worldwide attention. She claimed she inherited characteristics of the young man whose organs she received.

A Maine teenager's death in a 1988 motorcycle crash ended up giving life to Claire Sylvia of Hull. Over the years, Sylvia kept in touch with the family.

"She was a wonderful person," the teenager's mother said, fighting back tears in a telephone interview from her home in Saco. "As long as she was living it was as if my son was still alive. Now that she is gone, I know that my son is gone."

Sylvia said she developed unexplained cravings, such as a taste for beer, that she found out were traits of her donor.

"She was amazing," her daughter, Amara Cohen, said. "She was generous and caring. She was a great mother and grandmother. She went through a lot and she survived."

Sylvia was 47 when she learned she was dying from primary pulmonary hypertension.

"For a year or more she could only talk in a whisper and slowly," longtime friend Mary Kennedy of Cohasset said.

Kennedy first met Claire Sylvia in the late 1970s when she was giving dance lessons at her Hull home.

Following the heart-lung transplant, Claire Sylvia was back on her feet and vibrant as ever. She was a great believer in the supernatural and the spiritual, but she also had her two feet firmly on the ground, according to Kennedy.

"She had a quirky sense of humor. No matter how angry she got, she could always laugh herself out of it. She never held grudges."

Claire Sylvia, after living in Hull for 30 years moved to Florida. She became a best-selling author in 1997 with "A Change of Heart: A Memoir."

The book was published in 12 languages and made into a film, "Heart of a Stranger," starring Jane Seymour.

Claire Sylvia later promoted the need for more organ donors and appeared on the Phil Donahue and Oprah Winfrey television shows to talk about her experiences.

In 1998, she had additional health problems that led to her receiving a kidney from a former dance partner, who proved a match despite the two being unrelated.

Cohen said her mother had been living in a Brookline apartment while preparing to move to Linden Ponds, a Hingham retirement community.

The exact cause of death hasn't been determined although Claire Sylvia's daughter said her mother did have a blood clot on her lung, was coughing and feeling weak when she was admitted to the hospital. She was due to be released and go to a rehabilitation facility when she died.

Sylvia was also survived by two grandsons, a sister, and her son-in-law.

Doctor Deepak Chopra M.D. Celebrated author and television personality from the 1980s states, "This is a story that must be told and heard...a fascinating example of how cellular memory can outlive physical death."

Reference:*http://www.medicaldaily.com/can-organ-transplant-change-recipients-personality-cell-memory-theory-affirms-yes-2 http://www.patriotledger.com/x866753736/Organ-transplant-recipient-dies*

The late Claire Sylvia's book 'A Change of Heart' is available from Amazon Books

CHAPTER 5

Steve is a medical doctor... a General Practitioner from New South Wales. He lives with his wife and two daughters on the South Coast.

Steve has always had a healthy lifestyle and is a keen surfer so he and his family were shocked to find he had dilated cardiomyopathy (DCM) the heart muscle illness that sometimes leads to a heart transplant.

Doctor Steve tells his story.

"I was well until 2005 when I was diagnosed, or at least I had no idea I had severe dilated cardiomyopathy until I had an echocardiogram with our visiting cardiologist from Canberra (Australian Capital city.)

The year before I'd walked with a 20 kilogram plus pack on the South Coast track of Tasmania, one of the relatively hard walks in that State. I'd noticed that climbing over the Ironbound range I was struggling a bit.

Previously I'd loved climbing, but on this trip I struggled but man-

aged to complete it. In retrospect carrying my daughters upstairs to bed had also become more difficult.

My eldest was eight years of age and the youngest five.

You just put it down to getting older and being unfit.

Interestingly just before doing the Tasmania trip I'd had a respiratory tract infection that put an end to my plans to train up for the walk. Maybe that was the trigger, but I doubt it, seeing there were other subtle signs that I hadn't thought were important.

Anyhow, after that I had some vague chest pains that were brief and on the side of the chest. I'd had a colleague who had a malignant tumor in his chest which was diagnosed after he did his own Chest X-ray so I thought I should do a Chest X-ray.

The finding there was that I had cardiac enlargement. I wasn't too worried but thought it was a bit weird.

I certainly didn't expect that the next investigation would be so devastating.

In under a week the visiting cardiologist got me in to see him. The echocardiogram was bad news.

I was devastated and tearful, the grief compounded by my wife Robyn and I having two young girls. I'd gone to the appointment by myself so the drive along the Moruya River home to tell the news was one I'll never forget -usually a beautiful drive but my head was full of the diagnosis and the possible ramifications.

Dr O'Connor referred me to St Vincent's Hospital in Sydney for further assessment.

Pretty soon after that appointment with Professor Macdonald I was

Margot Maurice

referred on to have an implantable defibrillator inserted. **(An implantable cardioverter defibrillator (ICD) is a small device that's placed in the chest or abdomen.)**

I'd already started on Beta Blockers but they were knocking me for six. I think with the low heart rate I just had no energy. It's that old equation, Cardiac output equals heart rate by stroke volume and my stroke volume was shabby.

Going in for the ICD was nerve wracking. I don't think I've passed urine that frequently anytime in my life.

My life after the ICD stabilized a bit. In retrospect the first five or six years I was pretty stable and my functioning was maintained though I had to stop surfing our local river mouth break as the paddle against the incoming tide proved too much for me.

I had to stop bush walking. I wasn't allowed to carry a pack for fear the weight could damage the ICD leads. I kept working as a GP with hospital duties. Our local hospital has no physicians so as GPs we looked after the medical patients on the ward, did casualty and I continued to do anesthetics.

I backed off work a bit but really maybe only by 20%. I still traveled with the family but was a bit more wary of where we went in case things went pear shaped in the third world. I saw the Heart and Lung clinic at St Vincent's Hospital twice a year.

The echocardiograms didn't change. The hope that it was going to get better disappeared, but at least I wasn't getting worse either.

The echocardiograms showed a heart with very little action going on. It pretty much looked like a still picture, rather than an active pumping organ.

Looking back I'm amazed that the body can function despite such terrible organ performance. Kidney and liver failure is similar. It's not until things are really very bad that it becomes obvious-even for *an experienced health professional such as I. I had been a doctor for more than 20 years.*

Things got worse for me in late 2013, eight years after diagnosis. I got to a stage where I couldn't lie down comfortably or do any activity without feeling dizzy and or breathless. I'd look at the small lawn in front of my place and think of maybe doing the edges one day then the small patch of lawn the next. I'd been lucky that I hadn't had any hospital admissions but I'd had a couple of ventricular arrhythmia leading to two shocks. The latter of these resulted in a brief collapse and shocked my daughter more than me. I just got up and kept walking down the beach and she was very distressed.

One foot in front of the other, hour by hour, day by day. I really didn't hold out any hope of getting better. Certainly the prospect of transplantation was hardly on my radar.

I think when you are really sick you just see that deteriorating trajectory in front of you. I tended to not cling to some vague hope of a life, post transplant as it was so intangible and really so unlikely in my mind.

Anyhow my deterioration resulted in a transfer by air from the South Coast to St Vincent's in Sydney for stabilization on intravenous inotropic therapy (heart pump stimulators.)

It was only then after I had my first right heart catheter that Professor MacDonald and one of the surgeons said that I was going on the list. They tried to reassure me that I would get a heart in time but again I doubted it, particularly after coming home, as I was just feeling worse, losing weight with no appetite or energy.

I knew how difficult it was to get a heart, but knew having a family would help with my priority.

The work up was extensive requiring multiple trips to Sydney to see psychiatrists, the social worker, for all sorts of tests. It's all a blur really. It took over a month to get the work-up done ...then there was waiting.

*I was never offered a LVAD assist device (**A left ventricular assist device**, or **LVAD**, is a mechanical pump that is implanted inside a person's chest to help a weakened heart pump blood. Unlike a total artificial heart, the **LVAD** doesn't replace the heart. It just helps it do its job) and my awareness of these was only from meeting other transplant recipients and others on the wait list.*

Being five hours from Sydney may have been a factor with that. I had some medication alterations and there were some new medications coming out but I may have been a bit too far gone for them.

I was very fortunate getting a call for possible transplant within a month of going on the list.

I'll never forget the day. I'd been down to the beach. I kite surf and believe it or not I was still trying to do it. I was skilled at it and I'd pick my day. Not with strong winds and the sun had to be shining. I'd get a mate to carry my gear to the beach and help me launch. I'd use an electric pump to blow the kite up. Most of the effort is blowing up the kite and then it's just technique but I struggled after less than 10 minutes feeling nauseated from liver congestion with my right heart failing causing back pressure to my liver.

I collapsed on the beach dry retching and nauseated. My mate helped me backup and I headed home to bed to collapse.

I was always worried I'd get an arrhythmia whilst kiting and collapse and drown but the benefit to my psyche outweighed that small risk. I decided the benefit risk /discomfort ratio meant that would be my last kite.

Anyhow, I went to bed and to sleep in the middle of the day then received that call... a private number. I thought for sure it would be someone trying to sell me something and questioned whether I should answer the call. Then I remembered, I was on the waiting list.

Of course it was the Professor from St Vincent's calling. He told me they had a possible donor heart but it most likely had Takotsubo cardiomyopathy -a reversible disease of the heart caused by extreme stress. He was confident that the heart would recover and wanted me to come up for matching and assessment as to whether it would be suitable for me.

When you're put on the list they advise you, you may get called up a number of times without having transplant as you may not be a match or the heart may be found not to be suitable. There is also the possibility someone else has a higher priority. I went up with my mate after saying good bye to my girls telling them that I love them and reassuring them I'd be back tomorrow.

Anyhow, the heart was found to be suitable.

I remember being in casualty, having bloods taken and then the next thing is being in the anesthetic bay having an arterial line and peripheral line inserted.

I wasn't scared, just matter of fact. I'm a bit of a fate person. Whatever will be will be and stressing about it doesn't help anything.

My heart was transported using the new "heart in the box technology." This enabled the heart to be maintained beating and perfused with nutrients so it would be in better shape when transplanted.

In fact without this device, this heart would have been rejected as there was some thickening felt in one of the smaller coronary vessels.

Margot Maurice

The next thing I remember was waking up in ICU, sitting up with a tube down by throat unable to speak. The girls were there but I felt like a seal with the sounds I was making.

My stay in ICU had been more prolonged apparently because I'd been quite agitated when they wound down the sedation and they were concerned I may pull out my pacing wires.

I had a few more days in ICU due to bed block, then the ward for a month.

My post op recovery was complicated by the most vivid visual hallucinations involving the Grinch (believe it or not), Giant smurf-like creatures racing hot rods in a giant water park, scorched earth and watery seaweed creatures. It was totally bizarre. I knew they weren't real but as soon as the sun started to go down, my mind would produce these frightening, persistent scenes that gave me no prospect of rest.

I hardly slept for the first month. I think the hallucinations were caused by high dose steroids but possibly also the tacrolimus (tac) anti-rejection drug.

Post-transplant you have a regime of heart biopsies and I was very fortunate to only have low grade rejection levels, necessitating only small changes in medication doses.

I was very sensitive to some medications and had renal impairment that made dosing more tricky.

The other thing that amazes me is how easy it is to lose condition. I lost all my proximal muscles and my bum. I had quite marked peripheral swelling as my blood proteins were low. I needed high dose diuretics to gradually get rid of that, but above all that, my heart was beating like a trojan. No longer a still picture but an active beating healthy organ. What a sight to behold. I just cried tears of joy. My kidneys eventually improved.

Obviously, the feeling around transplant is strongly affected by the thoughts of someone else's loss of life and the grief of their family. I also thought often about how come I had the privilege to receive this heart, when others were still waiting. But I trusted that the specialists came to their decisions, using their own guidelines and I had no influence in it. Probably my catholic guilt also coming through.

I think my family were over the moon about the transplant as was I. I don't think we had any firm ideas about it before. The steroids made me a bit manic, hypomanic we call it in the trade and I adopted an alter ego who took to Instagram. I won't go into all that but it helped get us through the recovery phase, with laughter and a bit of craziness.

I pushed myself to get mobile, but just standing and then taking a step, was a huge challenge as I had lost so much strength and I think the drugs also affected my balance. But I pushed on doing laps of the ward, practicing walking heel to toe and doing repeated 'sit to stand' exercises. The physios only helped me with my first go on stairs which was terrifying and difficult, due to my muscle weakness. It was hard being away from family, but I would see them most weekends. In the end, I didn't want them coming up to visit every weekend, as it was throwing them out with their studies and leisure time.

I had the routine month in hospital. Blood tests and Chest X-rays most days. Drainage of a pleural effusion was my only surgical issue. The wound was remarkably pain free. Chest tubes are another story altogether.

My main problem was kidney impairment and my new heart was running too slowly, so I had to have the external pacer attached and be given ventolin, to try to speed the heart up. It gave you the shakes and it's interesting how tremor makes you feel frail. The problem with having the wires in, is that they ooze serous fluid continuously. (serous discharge is quite common after cardiac surgery a real mess,) and you need to be continually on intravenous antibiotics to prevent infection. I felt pretty "toxed" out on those. Anyhow eventually at the end of my stay, the pacing wires came out and at least I could have a proper shower, rather than a bed sponge. That was like heaven. I cried tears of joy.

Yes, hospitals are a bit like prison, when you can't leave the ward because your heart is being monitored continuously. The staff were fantastic - orderlies, nurses and doctors. St Vincent's is a fantastic institution. I can't thank the team enough.

I had another 2 months in Sydney, doing rehabilitation programs and having further biopsies and doctors' appointments. I got stronger and had the awesome support of a close family friend, who looked after me, feeding me delicious treats.

Eventually I got to go home and that was amazing, to be back home on the beautiful South Coast.

That winter was a challenge, as I felt the cold really easily and still couldn't get into the water -sports that I love...surfing, kite surfing, tennis and **sup** surfing. (There is a wide range of surfing **SUPs** from performance boards to all-rounders, so with help you can get into one of the most exciting parts of the sport. The Surf-specific Stand Up Paddleboard is more specialized than all-round Stand Up Paddleboard.)

Reference: how-to-surf-waves-on-your-sup

I had visits every four to six weeks that eventually dropped to six monthly. Now, I tend to fly up for the day, using the 'Isolated patients' scheme' to help cover some of the costs. My main other complication was a CMV infection. (**Cytomegalovirus infection** is a common herpes virus **infection** with a wide range of symptoms: from no symptoms to fever and fatigue (resembling **infectious** mononucleosis) to severe symptoms involving the eyes, brain, or other internal organs.)

I acquired this from the donor heart as I had never had exposure to it as a child. Luckily I never got really sick from that and it could be managed with antiviral medication.

From Spring on I went from strength to strength. I progressed back onto shorter and shorter surfboards once my chest discomfort settled and started the kite surfing season tentatively at first.

I was so much healthier than pre-transplant. I felt like the luckiest person on earth and still do really. It's such an amazing gift. So much good out of a tragedy. To be able to be here for my girls... it brings me to tears now. What can you say?

I started back at work initially just doing a journal club with the GP registrars, then some consulting and now I'm back doing hospital work (but not casualty shifts... I have too little ability to avoid infectious illness) and anesthetics.

I'm more than two years down the track. I'm on a stack of pills-low dose steroids, two other anti-rejection drugs plus calcium, magnesium and vitamin D. One antiviral, a cholesterol pill and aspirin plus on acid suppressor.

The other problem I had was burning pins and needles from the tacrolimus but that has settled gradually with dose adjustment and some mirtazapine.

My heart rate is still a bit slow but I don't need a pacemaker. I've traveled overseas a bit and plan a European trip later in the year. I *think the professor is happy with my progress. There are more tests planned. You do have an increased risk of coronary disease post transplantation in that transplanted heart but there's a program to monitor for that.*

The other thing I should comment on is the camaraderie and support you gain from other people on the journey pre and post- transplant. I maintain contact with many of them. I'm amazed at what other people have been through and the strength and determination of my fellow man.

I did suffer depression after the transplant. I think it was mid-winter and I just felt really agitated, unsafe and down.

It was pretty tough that winter. I think the likelihood of getting depression is increased by the effect of the steroids particularly having been manic for quite a while. I think the brain hormones are seriously messed with. I saw a counselor who said, "no wonder your feeling like that considering what you've been through." She said she didn't want to see me again which wasn't reassuring totally as I still felt unsettled. Things gradually improved as I moved onto the joys of summer on the South Coast, and long warm sunny days.

I think it was really ten to twelve months before I felt really well. Getting back to more work was really positive for me. Obviously it takes the focus off your own problems and that's great.

I struggled a bit with people always asking after my health but I know they cared about me. I think I just wanted to be a normal person rather than someone who had had a heart transplant. I struggle a bit when people focus on me and tend to shift it around pretty quickly by asking, "what can I help you with?"

I don't believe at all in the psychological changes one possibly gets from the donor heart. The heart is just a muscle and some nervous tissue which controls rate. I used to get a bit angry internally when people would ask about that but I realized that it's a common myth and I'd just deal with it with humor.

The other question is about who the donor was. That question would upset me too because I think, for me, it shows some lack of respect for the donor's family even though I know that was not the intent.

As part of the rehabilitation program recipients are encouraged to write an anonymous letter to the donor family. I found that hard to do but did so just under 12 months post - transplant. I know the family got the letter. I still feel their grief...

I think I've remained positive post - transplant. Before transplant I was a bit fatalistic. I don't think it would have helped me to be really upbeat and positive then as I felt pretty terrible. I'd still try to get out and do some activity. I wasn't depressed just realistic and a bit resigned to whatever would be would be...

I think we are so lucky to live in a country like Australia which has world class health facilities, despite our size. It's the luck of the draw that we don't struggle to have clean water, adequate food and shelter like so much of the world.

Since transplant, I took on the role of NSW contact for The Cardiomyopathy Association of Australia (Cardiomyopathy Australia) a position I'm still learning about.

I know having conversations with members helps them get through difficult times to some extent.

I want to get more involved with promoting organ donation too in order to give back something."

CHAPTER 6

This next story is Rhonda's. She lives in Western Australia and her illness started in 2002.

She went through a succession of surgeries and procedures over the following years and was fitted with a variety of aides in the hope they would improve her quality of life but she sank further and further down in health until finally she was placed on the heart transplant waiting list.

Rhonda's journey is quite different to some of the others I have used, as it emphasizes the truth, that every patient is different. Rhonda has battled on trying to care single handedly for her daughter who has Down Syndrome and is very reliant on her mother. She certainly is unable to fully understand how serious her mother's illness was going to affect the lives of each of them. *(Down syndrome (DS or DNS), also known as trisomy 21, is a genetic disorder caused by the presence of all or part of a third copy of chromosome 21.)*

Read on to get better understanding how tenacious Rhonda has been before, during and after her transplant.

Transplant...Life's Second Chance

Rhonda's story

"I was feeling very nauseated on the plane from Sydney to Perth in February 2002 but it wasn't a major problem, until my family and I were home and in bed. I had been traveling with my son, Jamie and my daughter Teoni.

About two a.m. I woke up feeling very panicky, gasping for air and having difficulty breathing. Sitting up and lying down were problematic, then all of a sudden, these feelings stopped and I slept until morning.

On waking I found it difficult getting out of bed, as any movement made me dizzy. Finally able to steady myself enough, I managed to dress and start the day. I soon realized any exertion caused a considerable lack of breath. I made an appointment with a doctor who was reasonably close to my home, as prior to this I had rarely had a need to see a doctor. Luckily, I was able to get an appointment for that Tuesday morning. Even though the surgery was only half a block away from my home, I had to drive as walking even ten meters, was like walking ten kilometers.

The doctor did some tests and asked for the results to be sent to him as soon as possible. He asked me to come back to see him later in the day and told me I would be his last patient for the evening.

A chest X-ray revealed pneumonia might be possible. Antibiotics were given and another appointment for the next day (Wednesday). This time a full blood test and another test. I cannot remember what it was and I was again asked to come back the next day (Thursday.) By now the night panics and breathlessness had not subsided and I had a strange feeling that something else may be suspected. On the Thursday the doctor made an appointment for a cardiac ultrasound for Friday morning and wanted the results as soon as possible and once again arranged for me to come back as his last patient that evening.

Margot Maurice

It was on the Friday he told me I had to go straight from the surgery to Fremantle hospital and arrangements were made for me to be met at the Emergency entrance by nursing staff. I remember asking could I go the next day so I could tell my son what was happening and to make arrangements to have my daughter cared for. Little did I know my ejection fraction was only nineteen and I didn't know what this figure represented. The doctor's response to my question was "definitely NO you cannot delay your emergency appointment."

Luckily my son who is a vegetarian and had been since he was five years of age had been trying to make me chicken soup so he was aware I was unwell. He was at home to help organize a few things and temporarily look after his sister and a good friend who lived nearby drove me to the hospital.

Staff met me and my first experience in the emergency department and a lifelong connection with hospitals, doctors, nurses, clinics, testing and various supplementary staff and services began. Memories of this time are rather hazy. I was left in the emergency ward's holding bay for a couple of days before being put in the only empty bed, way down the back with elderly people. I was stabilized and given a cocktail of tablets whilst in hospital and also given them to take with me when I went home. These were necessary to keep me alive. I was in hospital for approximately ten days and told I had dilated cardiomyopathy (DCM). At this time I knew very little about disease. Previous to this hospital admission, I'd only had the usual childhood problems such as appendicitis, measles and was a rather healthy 46 year old, who had to be coerced to take an analgesic.

A cardiologist was assigned to monitor me as an outpatient. These appointments at first were fortnightly then monthly then three monthly. My cardiologist decided I was to have an Intra Cardio Defibrillator (ICD) as he felt this was warranted. The electro-cardiac physiologist I was referred to confirmed an ICD was justified. I was reassured ICDs were safe and acted like an insurance policy and it was necessary to keep me alive. The device was fitted into my upper left side of my chest and an overnight stay in hospital was required.

I now had a device in my chest that would be my lifesaver on numerous occasions.

CHAPTER 7

Intra-Cardio Defibrillator (ICD - February 2006)

The ICD was inserted and felt as though it weighed much more than 200 grams. My chest felt as if a lump of lead had been inserted in the left side, and every night, it felt painful and extremely itchy. Every night I was extremely restless, scratching and rubbing the ICD area and decided that I'd have it taken out the next day. The next day was so busy, I was distracted enough until night time and this scenario would begin over again. This lasted for the first 8-10 days until the ICD site thankfully healed. The first six weeks after the ICD was inserted, I wasn't allowed to drive. Fortunately my friend Norm willingly put his life on hold and temporarily moved into my place to help me out. This was a godsend, as I didn't have any family in Western Australia.

By now I was very used to being on Marevan, a form of warfarin therapy which is an anticoagulant. This drug is commonly used in the treatment of heart problems to prevent clotting which can cause stroke and heart attack.

As warfarin can be affected by Vitamin K, certain other foods, some medications, and alcohol made it necessary to have regular blood tests to monitor my INR (International Normalized Ratio) levels. Ever since having DCM my INR levels were always erratic; which led to sometimes weekly, fortnightly or monthly blood tests to check my levels and adjust the dosage accordingly.

There were a few times I went into hospital; for 1-2 nights because of my ICD. Once I remember it fired 2-3 times in the Emergency Department and they pressed the resuscitation button. Doctors and nurses came from everywhere. After a transfer to Coronary Care Unit, a nurse Michelle was assigned to me all night.

I know I had pulmonary oedema (fluid on the lungs) a few times, Ventricular Tachicardia (VT) an erratic heart rhythm in the ventricular and bradycardia slow heart rate. My heart would mostly go into VT (despite being on long-term Amiodarone medication to stabilize heart rhythms) After the 2nd time I could tell when I was going into VT. I'd immediately press my button, ask for a nurse I knew would come straight away. And believe me, I am sure an arrest was averted once or twice because of this. I remember a trainee doctor came in to see me afterwards and asked me what I thought would have happened. When I told him, he looked at me kind of cross eyed. I still wonder if he believed me that day.

My (ventricular assist device) **VAD** *is a mechanical pump that's used to support heart function and blood flow in people who have weakened hearts. The device takes blood from a lower chamber of the heart and helps pump it to the body and vital organs, just as a healthy heart would.*

VAD was inserted before transfer from Intensive Care Unit (ICU), to Coronary Care Unit (CCU) and even in my hallucinatory state, I wanted a cup of tea. As soon as I woke up, I asked for a cup of tea.

Margot Maurice

All day long I kept pestering every two minutes and my frustrated nurse kept saying, she would make one when she could. As soon as her shift finished she made my cup of tea; the exact moment it was brought over, the orderlies came to take me to CCU!

Plasmapheresis *is a method of removing blood plasma from the body by withdrawing blood, separating it into plasma and cells, and transfusing the cells back into the bloodstream. It is performed especially to remove antibodies, in treating autoimmune conditions.*

I guess this was done about 12 times. 2-3 times as an outpatient, then pre-transplant and again in the coronary care unit. The procedure takes approximately 45 minutes and I became extremely cold and shivered each time. Once I had five blankets and was still cold! The other times a very light nylon plastic electric air blanket was placed over me, then an ordinary blanket on top. The air blanket blows out fine streams of warm air, which was absolutely comforting.

Approximately a year later April 2007, Norm who regularly stayed at my house if he needed to come to the city, found me on the laundry floor. My ICD for the first time, had shocked my heart and I had collapsed. He immediately bundled my very distraught daughter, Teoni, into his car and took me into Royal Perth Hospital (RPH) Emergency Department (ED), where I showed the staff a card which I had been instructed to always carry with me. I was given that card when I had the ICD inserted and I was taken immediately to Emergency Department resuscitation area. At this moment, my ICD went off twice more! My blood test results came back that I was very low in Vitamin K and Magnesium. My ICD was tweaked and the next day I was allowed home.

To prepare us for any problem, Royal Perth Hospital (RPH) had given us a lot of ICD information and held an ICD meeting every 6 months. The meetings consisted of a guest speaker, a clinical nurse or nurse practitioner and a Guidant representative. This was followed by a Question and Answer session. These were extremely informative and the morning tea was yummy. Life went along rather well, until one Tuesday night a few months later.

Luckily, once again Norm was visiting us. This night, I remember not feeling very well and asked Norm to pick Teoni up from drumming classes. Norm remembers hearing a 'gunshot' noise as he returned and walked through the door. He found me extremely dazed, staring glazed into the air. He said I had to go with him in the car and I remember following him, as if I was in a trance.

Meanwhile all Teoni wanted was her dinner! Again at RPH I bypassed the reception and was taken once again to resuscitation, where a nurse and cardiac registrar doctor stayed by my side, until I was transferred to the Coronary Care Unit (CCU). Each time I was admitted, a routine blood test was done, an Intravenous (IV) line inserted, an Electrocardiogram (ECG) and a heart monitor hooked up. Then there was as well, the usual Blood Pressure machine, chest x-rays, oxygen and whatever else was deemed necessary at the time.

One memory I have of this admission is not having any clothes, hair brush or other toiletries with me. I would buy some when the Red Cross trolley came around.

When it finally arrived, I had some money out ready, but when it did come, the Red Cross woman stopped the trolley outside my door with her back turned away. She was talking to someone! I was on bed rest and unable to speak very loudly- and there was no way of getting her attention. She didn't look around when she finished talking but continued with the trolley to other rooms!

Margot Maurice

In September 2007 on my ex-husband's birthday, my son Jamie fractured his thoracic vertebrae T5 and T6. Teoni and I flew to Melbourne as Jamie had moved there six months prior, with his girlfriend, to study at Deakin Uni, as he was concerned about his future.

Fortunately he didn't have any spinal injury except for the fracture and was discharged a few days later with minimal movement and the reassurance that his girlfriend would care for him. Teoni and I decided to stay a few more days until Jamie's birthday later that month. We took him some birthday treats in the afternoon. Teoni and I planned to return to WA the day after.

Near Flinders Street railway station about 11am, I began to feel my heart pound slightly and my breathing increase. I still kept shopping, as I was a little bit frightened, plus wasn't sure what was happening and hoping it would STOP! In the supermarket it became much worse and uncontrollable until I had to sit on the ledge where the milk was. The staff were worried and asked for someone's phone number they could dial to come to pick me up.

The only number I was able to retrieve before I dropped my mobile on the floor was Jamie's girlfriend. Fortunately Jamie was with her and I asked them to immediately call an ambulance. By the time the ambulance arrived, I was gasping for air and had no strength to move or speak. All I remember was the ambulance driver asking me "is that your daughter?" and then telling Teoni to follow them.

The next I was aware of anything was later in the night. I was in a hospital bed near the nurses' station, with an extremely exhausting breathing apparatus strapped to my face. It was inflating my lungs at regular intervals. After, I was to learn how critical I was. The machine was known as a **continuous positive airway pressure (CRAP)**, *and is a treatment that uses mild air pressure to keep the airways open.* **CRAP** *typically is used by people who have breathing problems, such as sleep apnea.* **CRAP** *also may be used to treat preterm infants whose lungs have not fully developed. This was necessary to keep me alive along with the plethora of tubes I had around me.*

The next day I was told I had been admitted to St Vincent's Public Hospital Melbourne, after being in Emergency for about 5 hours.

Looking back, I have a feeling this was the first time I had to be resuscitated and found my jumper had been cut down the back for me to be treated. The nurses had put a mattress on the floor next to me for Jamie to rest when he visited, and Teoni was found crying in the Emergency corridor. She went home that night with Jamie. A very dear friend of mine and also Teoni's godmother had arranged for her to stay with them, until we knew what was going to happen. Two of my sisters were on their way from NSW. Apart from everyone telling me what a nice room I had and the view was great, which I had no interest in, what happened for the next few days were rather blurry?

I do remember, this was my first introduction to daily fluid reduction of 1200 mls which included ALL types of fluids! Ice, icy poles and frozen oranges became very important to me and I felt continuously thirsty. Another memory, is the activity was continuous. My family and friends continued to be very helpful and attentive. I think about day five, I was allowed to go downstairs for a coffee. About day six I was told I wasn't allowed to go back to Perth for at least 6-8 weeks. It was arranged for Teoni to fly back to Perth and stay with her boyfriend's family, until I came home. In retrospect I haven't the foggiest who paid for or made arrangements for this flight!

About day 8 – 10 I was discharged and stayed with my sisters for 2 nights before they went home. I continued in Melbourne staying at a friend's house. As she was working, she told me I could have her car each day, after driving her to work. I was to pick her up after she finished work. This was handy, as I had a few medical appointments to attend as well as some shopping. Six to eight weeks later I was finally told I could come back to WA.

Margot Maurice

Arriving in Perth, surprisingly Norm had driven from his home in Quairading (a small country town about 250 kilometers away) to meet me. He had bought milk, food and other items for when I came home. He had also decided he was staying at my house for a while until I recuperated. Little did he know he was not going to return to Quairading for many years. Teoni came home, Norm stayed to make sure I was all right and life went on as usual for a while.

A couple of weeks later, a meeting was arranged with disability services to discuss a plan for Teoni's future. Norm said he'd stay for the meeting and leave to go home to Quairading when it finished. Teoni and I, together with Norm, Teoni's dad Steve, her boyfriend Owen, his mum Sue, and a disability worker attended.

Half way through the meeting I began again to breathe rapidly and my heart was racing. As this progressed I stopped the meeting to have a break thinking it may help. The disability worker asked if I needed anything and I said "an ambulance" ... she then proceeded to tell me she'd make me a cup of tea. Norm appeared from the loo and straightaway said he was taking me to hospital. I shook my head and said 'an ambulance' before I fell on the floor unconscious. On the way to the hospital I briefly woke up and the ambulance officer asked me how I felt? I remember saying "as if I'm going to die." He replied "you are not going to die" then once again I was unconscious. I also have a vague memory of coming around slightly and wondering what was happening before realizing someone was pounding on my chest. Obviously and scarily someone was doing CPR! Norm was told if I survived that night in the Intensive Care Unit, I'd probably survive and be transferred from Fremantle hospital to the Coronary Care Unit (CCU) at RPH. I remember that trip, being transferred to RPH. I had to be accompanied by a doctor, 2 nurses and an ambulance officer driving. It was the bumpiest ride I'd ever been on! Thankfully Norm stayed at my place and Sue had taken Teoni home with her. I was to be in hospital. Steve, my ex-

husband who is Teoni's Dad, went back to Bunbury by himself.

At RPH emergency department I was greeted by Trevor, the CCU Nursing Unit Manager and that's all I remember until sometime after various tests were done in CCU. My weight at this stage was 58 kg, my BP 70/40. Again my memory of this time is very vague. I was told it was too dangerous for me to go home as my heart was constantly going from beating reasonably to VT. I was in a room opposite the nurses' station with the usual IVs, a heart monitor, BP cuff, and a very attentive nursing staff coming and going and checking any changes at all times of the day and night.

All I remember from this time is lots of being poked and prodded, and the Advanced Heart Failure and Cardiac Transplant Service (AHFCTS) team, that consisted of one or two cardiologists, the cardiology registrar, the pre-transplant, post-transplant nurse practitioners (NP)), the Ventricular Assist Device (VAD), an assistant Clinical Nurse Consultant and a student cardiac nurse or another nurse coming each morning. On the 2nd morning they came and suggested I needed a VAD! My reply was "a what?"

CHAPTER 8

Ventricular Assist Device (VAD) (November 2007)

I was to learn a VAD is a mechanical machine, which is a bridge to transplant that acts as an artificial heart. Mine consisted of a small titanium pump implanted into the heart with a cord (drive line) going into the stomach. One end of the cord is connected to the pump whilst the other is connected outside the body to a small controller (a type of computer and data collection device) with batteries which powered the pump inside the heart. All this fitted neatly into a bag about the size of a video recorder bag.

The next time I saw the **Advanced Heart Failure and Cardiac Transplant Services (NP AHFCTS) Team** *they weren't sure which type of VAD would be beneficial for me and I wasn't sure I really wanted one. It was explained I had 2 choices; a VAD or the alternative; basically I could choose to live or die!*

The 2 types of VAD were:

1. *The large bulky non portable type where the patient has to stay in hospital until a donor heart is available or*

2. *The new portable version (as above) which was currently being trialed before approval. It was a worldwide trial of 50 VADS with* *various hospitals in selected countries and RPH was part of this trial.*

The trial was being run by an American based company and this was the first portable VAD to gain approval worldwide. The difference between this VAD and previous VADS was that a patient could go home with this VAD insitu and live a reasonably normal life in the community. The implant of this VAD was conditional, inasmuch as the patient wasn't allowed to drive and required a full time live-in carer who was entitled to receive the fortnightly government Carer Allowance. Norm at first was rejected for this allowance because his regular address was Quairading. For some reason someone at Centrelink couldn't grasp that he was now staying in Perth. It was approved after the section manager became involved.

As I wanted to live, a VAD was inevitable. The idea of being a guinea pig in a trial frightened me very much! Lots of information and explanation was given to me and a former VAD recipient Matt came in to show me how a VAD worked. This was extremely encouraging and allayed some fears I had. Since I was so thin and weak, the cardiology team wanted to wait until I had built up some strength and condition before inserting a VAD. I had to hold my nose to drink the protein drinks I was supposed to have. The smell and taste of these drinks was vile! The following Wednesday I had open heart surgery and a VAD was implanted into my heart. After surgery the next few days were not at all pleasant. I certainly wasn't prepared for what had happened. Lying in bed, dribbling, unable to move, cough or turn without my whole body hurting was extremely harrowing. The hallucinations lasted for days until I realized that's what had been happening. It was at this point I became aware and receptive enough to be involved in my recovery. The only good parts were the warm lux daily bed baths that felt so good. It took a few weeks to recover because when I had been admitted to hospital, my condition was extremely life threatening.

The next few weeks proved to be challenging for me, Norm and everyone involved; getting used to having a VAD and the care needed. My VAD was the 7th for RPH and 48th in the world. I was assigned the number 007 and decided to call my VAD Gucci. As these VADs were relatively new most of the nurses and staff hadn't seen one before, it seemed everyone had to learn together.

Having a VAD involved a few changes, plus being plugged into electricity each time I was in bed at night when home, but powered with batteries controlling the pump when out and about. A daily dressing was required for the drive line site into the tummy, changing batteries when necessary, a daily weight check to monitor fluid retention, carrying another bag ALL the time. That had spare batteries, then being aware of problems and, what to do plus general daily care. Having a shower or bath wasn't allowed because the VAD had an electric current. Teoni wasn't allowed to come home and fortunately Sue said Teoni could stay with her. I was so grateful. Norm had said he'd stay in Perth until a heart donor was available, hallelujah! The next few weeks in hospital were spent recovering, having many cardiac ultrasounds, blood tests and meeting the cardiac dietician. Then there was a social worker, psychologist and many allied cardiac staff.

Hair washing became a major saga. I soon learned to say I was a vegetarian as the food smelt and tasted yuk! Norm came in daily and gradually learned what was expected of him as my carer. Part of my recovery involved having physiotherapy at first then following a line around the ward.

I walked around as many times as I felt comfortable and then going to the cardiac gym daily. My first attempt at the gym was outside for the first time and was a god send, even though it took forever to hop out of bed and into a wheelchair. It was even longer once at the gym as I had to hop onto a bike and complete 2 minutes exercise. All in all because I was so breathless and it hurt so much I must have been away at least an hour to do 2 minutes exercise! Twice at some stage my blood pressure (BP) was 70/40 and I had to go to clinic because I was dehydrated and had to be reassessed. The gym was to become the best support and a rather social occasion.

Unbeknown to me at the time, the lady (Ceri) I mentioned earlier, had been seen walking around the ward crying when I was admitted. She was upset after being told she needed a VAD as a bridge to heart transplant. She had no previous heart disease history and had presented to her local GP a week before with pneumonia. Her VAD (number 50 and the end of the trial) was implanted the week after mine. Her recovery was much less eventful.

We became extremely close friends. Coincidentally, whatever Ceri did or needed, so did I and vice versa. One day at the gym both of us were dehydrated and had low blood pressure and both of us collapsed onto the gym floor at the same time. Colin who also had a VAD was with Ceri and I going somewhere when he went into VT and alarms kept going off. I was in a wheelchair but had to let Colin have it and he was taken to clinic. Ceri and I were half through the test when both of us also went into VT. All 3 of us had low Vitamin K and magnesium levels. Both Ceri and I were transferred to the same room one day and then had an IV potassium drip going. IV potassium is cruel as it has to run extremely slowly and stings at the IV site along the vein. These coincidences continued until we were discharged. Even now we both watch what happens to each other and amazingly it is very similar. We've often checked with other heart recipients about the same time as us and they're not having the same experiences. It is a rather disconcerting phenomena. Ceri was discharged about a week before me and I was allowed to go home on Christmas Eve. Both of us were given more information about VADS, an instruction booklet about what to do and not do, an emergency after hours paging number. We were told we were to stay within an hour's drive of Perth. This procedure can be a major disruption to the person's life. Ceri had come from Busselton 2.5 hours south of Perth. Ceri and her husband (carer) were not able to go home until Ceri had her heart transplant. Because both of them worked. Their income was affected, plus they had to find accommodation whilst in Perth for an unspecified time. Norm on the other hand, although disrupted from his daily country living in Quairading, was retired and as my carer had accommodation at my place.

Christmas turned out to be a great day; Teoni came home for the day and a few friends brought lunch over. After Christmas the reality of having a VAD and the limitations was rather daunting. Norm and I soon settled down into a routine for regular VAD checkups and in preparation to be listed for a heart transplant. I was expected to go to the RPH cardiac gym 3 times a week, the VAD clinic, a dietician and a psychologist weekly. Then there was a psych test and numerous other tests including CT scans, VO2, chest x-ray and a full MRI on other days. RPH soon became a safe haven and for the first 3 months we spent almost every weekday waiting on the same chairs for hours outside the AHFCTS clinic. We became very familiar with many cardiac patients, all the staff on the 4th floor plus the staff at the coffee shop. At one stage the RPH coffee shop became our regular meeting place for all our friends and visitors.

A month after being discharged with my VAD, I saw the Director of Cardiopulmonary Transplantation Mr Rob Larbalestier and given the 3rd degree about what can and cannot be done whilst listed for cardiac transplantation.

I told him I needed a stiff scotch before I agreed and he told me he'd need one too if he was in my situation and it would do me the world *of good!*

Having an aversion to scotch I was listed for a heart transplant without ever having that scotch.

I was given a special pager to carry with me all the time. The pager would buzz to alert me to contact the AHFCTS when a suitable donor heart was available. There were 8 people in Perth currently listed for a transplant. About 3 months later I received news that the VADs were approved and freely available; not only as a bridge to transplant but also as a mechanism to end of life for suitable patients. Joe who was number 3 VAD at RPH during the trial and is the longest living VAD recipient in the world which was 8 years in July 2016. Sadly patients after Ceri who would have benefited with a VAD couldn't have one until the VADs were approved.

*A few days before I was discharged, my sister Elaine came over to WA for a month to visit and to give Norm a much needed break. He was able to go back to Quairading to check on his home, mail and other things. Elaine learned about the VAD, low flows occur with the heart arrhythmias: usually caused by dehydration, low Vitamin K or low magnesium as much as I remembered. Elaine learned how to do my dressing and all the bits and pieces pertaining to being a VAD carer! She provided respite for Norm and much needed family reassurance for me. Every day I felt so much better and it wasn't long before I felt **so** good. I hadn't felt this well for years, like my old normal self! Although I had to have a daily dressing, do a daily weight, a clexane (subcutaneous anti-coagulant) injection, weekly/daily checkups/tests, I also had to carry a bag around and battery bag everywhere I went, then I had to have a carer by my side almost 24/7, and my VAD side hurting constantly as if bruised. In spite of all these, I felt fantastic and it actually was an enjoyable time for me.*

Margot Maurice

What we required was given freely by the AHFCTS, dressing packs, bio patches, mepilex, saline, gauze, everything I needed for my dressings and to be comfortable. Any and every complaint small or large was taken seriously. Apart from a few cardiac ultrasounds, iron infusions, and x-rays, overall my VAD experience was reasonably uneventful. At one stage I had a slight infection which is one of the most feared complications of any operation especially post VAD. The VAD drive line is a portal between the inside and outside of the body. As the line travels directly to the heart any infection has the potential to affect the heart which I've heard is extremely difficult to treat. This infection was treated with clindamycin (used to treat serious infections) 150 mg for 2 weeks and a special silver sulphur dressing around the drive line.

There were a few obstacles to overcome. I had to be close to electricity at all times to recharge the batteries. Changing batteries became second nature. An alarm would sound each time a battery was low. Whilst in bed, I had a longer cord that plugged into a socket, therefore a VAD is classified as life support. This enables an electricity supplement and to be emergency listed. The following winter whilst in bed with my Gucci VAD, I managed to somehow short out my electric blanket! Ambulance stations had to be notified. I was required to wear a stretchy belt around my waist to keep the drive line in place and stable. Bathing wasn't really allowed because electricity is involved, so the first 3 months was awkward. After that I devised a way to shower and wash my hair properly This was simply by putting a hook over the top of the shower rail and hanging the VAD up so no water got in. Another problem was having someone with me every minute of the day. Not being allowed to drive, go for a coffee, or do anything alone.

A few days after being home about 20 boxes of Sustagen other protein drinks arrived on my doorstep. The RPH dietician said I had to drink one with every meal. Drinking these drinks was such an ordeal, I packed all of the boxes into Norm's car and gave them to the homeless. Another memory was going to the airport one evening and being asked several times to put my VAD on the x-ray machine. In the end, I convinced security to let me through, as my VAD and I were attached. Once I accidentally pulled out the wrong lead which was the critical alarm, and you only have three seconds to put it back in. Thankfully I managed to do that.

*At the checkups, the technicians did a reading. This was a printout of everything that had occurred all day every day. With any alarm or problem, the VAD team had to be alerted, therefore even if you didn't feel like letting them know, they would find out. There were no secrets the VAD team **knew** it all. One night I went to the casino with Norm. He thought I had my battery bag and I thought he did. After a frantic search, someone tapped him on the shoulder. The security guy we spoke to at the door had it and thankfully remembered us. The fear of someone thinking the bag held a camera and grabbing it, was always in the back of my mind. Having to carry the VAD around all the time was boring and a nuisance at times.*

The following August, late one night, a donor heart was available. I was paged and called into RPH. There are some cross matching tests that can only be done at this time. I learned that the time was NOW, because my antibody count was extremely high and that increases the possibility of massive antibody rejection. I was to come back the next day to have it explained and Ceri was called in for her transplant.

CHAPTER 9

*HEART TRANSPLANT **(12 September 2008)***

A strange sound Friday afternoon September 11, 2008 at Chapman was my heart transplant pager beeping. Of all places to be, Norm and I were at a local hotel. Norm, who rarely drinks alcohol, had felt like a beer. Luckily Norm had only one beer and I hadn't anything to drink. Clumsily I called the AHFCTS and was told to come into RPH NOW! We hurriedly left the hotel and at the car realized I'd left my bag on the counter and had to go back to get it. We went home to grab an already prepared bag, containing the basics needed in hospital. I also remembered my VAD batteries to take with us and we headed off in peak hour traffic. It felt extremely surreal. On my way to Royal Perth Hospital (RPH) I called my son Jamie who was in Tasmania and my sister Elaine in New South Wales (NSW) to let them know what was happening.

At RPH we were met by the AHFCTS nurse Sharon who was on call and we were ushered into a small room. Here she explained what was going to happen. As I'd previously had preliminary pre-transplant tests the month before, they were almost certain the heart would be a match for me. We also knew I had to have plasma pheresis (process in which plasma is separated from the cells.) Plasma can contain antibodies that attack the immune system. A machine removes the affected plasma and replaces it with good plasma) prior to transplant. This was the reason why I couldn't have the transplant before and is when they determine that plasma pheresis is necessary. It took approximately an hour before it was set up. I knew what to expect as this would be my second of many. The process took several minutes and I was to put my hand up if I felt any affects. 42 minutes into my second plasma pheresis I felt like all the blood had suddenly drained from my body and put my hand up just before passing out. I have no memory of what happened next. Norm told me later when I was talking, had a shower, and dressed for theater, that I was co-operative until I went to the operating theater (OT).

*My first vague memories after OT was I could **hear** voices and a radio. After an indefinite time I realized the people talking were possibly nurses and that I was in a bed lying on my back, totally unaware of what was or had happened. I gathered it was a radio that was going on and off... that the voices were around most of the time and my thoughts were mostly hallucinations. I have an unclear memory of two orderlies coming in one night to roll me over. Although they didn't realize I could hear them, they still told me who they were and what they were doing. They were also talking to the nurse in my room about what was happening. I **think** she told them they would be back for me soon as I wouldn't make it through the night. My silent reply was "hang on, you're talking about me and I'm not going anywhere."*

As I began to wake up from my induced coma, I gradually became more aware of my surroundings and the radio seemed my only source of stimulation. When it was turned off I really wished someone would turn it back on.

I struggled to put together where I was and what had happened and recall that when I opened my eyes I saw two of my sisters Elaine and Kaye dancing by my bed and Norm holding my hand talking to me. There wasn't any way to let them know I could see them and knew who they were. I was aware I still had all the tubes in and I presumed I was still being ventilated as well as having a catheter, central line, oxygen and goodness knows what else. I was slipping in and out of consciousness and naturally not very lucid.

Over the next few days/weeks I saw my sisters and Norm come in together and most late evenings my son Jamie would come by himself or with some friends. One of his friends had dyed pink hair which I thought was amazing because this was the first color I'd seen for ages. Another evening when he came to see me, he was with a friend, Alisha and both were dressed up. He explained to me that they were going to a wedding as friends were getting married. My mind changed it to, **Jamie** *was marrying* **Alisha**. *I thought at the time it was odd, but okay. A couple of weeks later when I was able to congratulate him, he thought it was hilarious. The couple from the house where he was going to house sit while they went on a honeymoon, were* **those** *being married.*

Lying on that bed in an ICU private room, I would often look out into the main open area and wonder why the doctors were doing experiments over there on the other patients. Often my eyes would follow the nurse around the room, trying to work out what she was doing. When I **could** *and* **did** *turn my head, she reprimanded me. I haven't the foggiest idea how long I was there, how long I slept, whether it was night or day. I do remember thinking the longer I lie here, the longer it's going to take me to recover.*

In my mind at the time my recovery consisted of having the endotracheal tube out, (occurring within or performed by way of the trachea an endotracheal tube.) sitting up, pulling a tissue from a tissue box, having a BIG cough then I'd be okay. I do know it was boring and mostly not stimulating.

To regress to what I have been told happened is; I was the first patient in WA to have a heart that would not beat. My donor heart came from Adelaide and the plane encountered some turbulence so it arrived later than expected. My donor heart was out of the body for too long. Because of this I required extra corporeal membrane oxygenation (ECMO), was in an induced coma on life support. ECMO is usually only used during the operation but because of my heart being problematic I needed to stay on ECMO indefinitely. The other problem was I had massive antibody and antigen rejection. Then continued ECMO coupled with the rejection. No-one knew how I would be when I woke up nor what to expect.

*Nearly seven years later, I'm still unsure of any details. I asked the cardiologist in charge of AHFCTS what happened and his reply was "you don't want to know." Sometime later when I saw him, he was extremely surprised at how I was going and told me I was definitely the most difficult person they've had to treat and although he loves his job, it is people like me that are a difficult case but **do** make it, that make his job that much more rewarding.*

Apparently ECMO is only recommended for four days, only because of the risk of brain damage and as my chest was still open there was, in my case, the additional risk infection. They began seriously considering turning off my life support. I am told the doctor who was second in charge of ICU was rather insistent my life support be turned off as there wasn't any hope. Hallelujah, the AHFCTS cardiologist in charge and doctor in charge of ICU wanted to wait longer.

My heart had a very faint beat that afternoon!

Now, so I have been told, they turned something down (presumably life support) for a couple of minutes to see how I'd respond. Then it was 20 minutes until my heart began to beat on its own, then life support was turned off. That evening I was taken back to OT for my chest to be closed. Apparently, everyone went from being extremely worried to extremely happy. The endo tracheal tube seemed to remain in the same position for so long and was extremely uncomfortable. I think the doctor in charge of ICU came every day to let me know when they were taking it out but seemed to prolong doing so for days.

My sisters have told me since, I was blown up like a balloon and almost unrecognizable and told me I had machines and tubes everywhere. There were three people in the room the first few days. An ICU nurse and two technicians attending the ECMO and life support.

My chest was still open with blood everywhere and there was a type of glad wrap covering it.

Si-an, the cardiac registrar was on the phone to Melbourne for about 20 hours; finding out information, as I was the first ever in WA with a transplanted heart that wouldn't beat. They said, some people came on the 2nd or 3rd day and everyone was told they couldn't go inside to visit.

All the blinds were pulled down so no-one could see inside. These medical and technical people were inside for a long long time. Someone said they were taking photos of me. I'd signed so many papers that I hadn't the foggiest why ... I guess it was for some research material.

I was also told that Norm spent a lot of time at church and had recessional prayers said for me. He also wrote out prayer sheets to give out and asked everyone to pray for me.

I remember Norm often holding my hand and it often felt very hot. I presume I had a temperature at that time. I remember my son Jamie holding my hand one day when I was awake but I still couldn't talk, he told me he loved me and I was the most beautiful mother and the best mum he had!

The support I had was tremendous, as apart from Jamie who had come up from Tasmania, my two sisters (Elaine and Kaye) came the Tuesday after and Norm's son Sean flew down from the mines on extended leave to support his dad. Neither of them knew if I was going to be alive when they arrived.

Months later Jamie told me he'd actually said his goodbye to me as the doctors had told everyone it was touch and go but the possibility of me surviving was extremely unlikely. It was a godsend as was the cardiac surgeon, AHFCTS team, the ICU doctor in charge and staff.

This is all the memory I have of ICU and don't even remember being transferred to the Coronary Care Unit (CCU).

CHAPTER 10

POST-TRANSPLANT

Apparently because I had survived ICU and made it to CCU I was dubbed the 'Miracle Lady.' Miracle or no miracle, it all felt rather surreal and I felt numb, couldn't concentrate to watch television or read anything. I was extremely irritable and tired. Even more disappointing and surprising was I couldn't pull a tissue from a tissue box nor cough like I thought would make me well, whilst in ICU.

I was still having a cocktail of morphine based analgesia which still not only made me hallucinate but also be extremely tired. All I did in between procedures was sleep and dribble. I was totally floppy: I couldn't walk, couldn't talk, and could hardly move! There were still tubes and machines everywhere.

Fortunately I have a nursing background which helped me have an overall understanding what was going to happen and what was happening. The okay part was previously having had a VAD, it had paved the way for me to know the hospital routine, the ward and the nurses. This familiarity and friendliness helped a lot. I was in a single room over from the nurses' station and it was set up to be as comfortable as possible. My sisters and Norm would read my cards *for me, write out what day it was, any changes, my medications and any messages on a whiteboard on the wall in front of my bed. I was **completely** reliant on other people. It wasn't much fun ... didn't like it at all.*

My day would begin when a junior doctor came to take blood gases ... not an easy task after the plethora of blood tests I'd already had. It meant my veins had often collapsed numerous times and still do. A daily ECG and routine observations (BP, temperature) were done. I had a heart monitor, IV and oxygen saturation thing on full time. Later a daily soothing lux sponge bath felt absolutely luxurious and the best part of the day.

In those early days I had to have a very strong prophylactic drug called valganciclovir ((CMV) which is an anti-viral and anti Cytomegalic Virus (CMV) which has to be taken orally with food. My tablets were crushed or mixed into an icy pole and taken any which way I could get them from my mouth to my tummy. There were too many of them and were yuk, yuk, yuk! This is one of the reasons my sisters and Norm would try to make me eat meals. I would clench my teeth and refuse. Food was not appealing at all: the smell, the taste, the sight was YUK! Fruit smoothies, protein drinks and Sustagen were introduced to my diet. I had to hold my nose and drink as much as I could in one breath because they all tasted vile! Then the AH-FCTS team would do their rounds to discuss what's next, plus joke with me, knowing I could not talk therefore couldn't reply. These doctors and nurses were great. I was still on IV prednisolone and felt nauseated, short tempered, hyper-agitated and extremely itchy all over!

It wasn't long before physio began. The first few times I walked or tried to, was on a very tall walking frame which I flopped around on whilst being pushed around. I had someone walk beside me, another person pushing a wheelchair behind me in case I fell.

Visitors were now allowed, although limited to who and how many could come at once and for how long. Visitors were okay depending on how close I felt to them and if they just popped in it was okay. Otherwise they became a nuisance because I had NO energy, couldn't talk, looked like a blown up balloon and tried to stay awake to be polite when all I wanted to do was sleep.

After my sister Kaye went home, Elaine and Norm settled into a routine of coming each day to sit with me. This was mostly good and comforting to know someone cared enough to do this. They'd help do small chores, attend to me and generally be there as much as they could.

*Each day they'd write up anything new on the whiteboard, try to encourage me to eat, feed me my meals and do what they could. I remember my first hair wash in bed and Elaine helped the two or three nurses. Previously my hair had felt like dirty straw. It felt **soooo** good to have clean hair again. Thankfully I had done the Leukemia Big Hair Shave the previous March and so had short hair as I cannot imagine having my waist length hair during this time.*

The first few days or weeks were a blur. My legs were still so oedematous, I thought they would explode. They were painfully sore even to touch lightly, I had to literally pick them up as best I could to change their position. I felt as though I belonged in an African game park, my legs looked like they belonged to an elephant. My sternum still hurt a lot and holding a pillow close to my chest was still necessary. I couldn't cough or sneeze. My speech and movement was almost non-existent therefore I didn't progress. I was still very weak and anything I did, as much as I tried, my recovery rate took a very long time. I couldn't squeeze anyone's hand when asked and was continually pestered to walk or at least try, even though I still couldn't stand up by myself. Day by day I could raise my arms a little bit more than the day before. Just trying to take off or put on my PJ top was a major effort and would take forever. A few of the nurses were getting irritable with me and dubbed me as being lazy. My progress was extremely slow. I thought most of the nurses expected too much from their patients; some would expect the patient, including me to do everything by themselves, though it wore me out dreadfully. Often the nurses would abruptly tell me not to talk as they couldn't hear nor understand me! One nurse who had nursed me in ICU surprisingly gave me hope, said she couldn't believe I was the same person as before as I looked so different now. Elaine was also becoming irritable with me, as much as she tried to encourage me I still wouldn't/couldn't try. Luckily Norm said I was usually determined to try and there must be something wrong. Elaine paid a couple of days of TV for me, a friend brought in audio reading books, another a puzzle book, none of which I could concentrate sufficiently on to do, or had any interest in doing.

Russi became my usual physio. Each day he'd come and ask me to go for a brief walk. Everyday I'd say I didn't want to! Then he would say he'd come back after he'd seen another patient. He'd get the same reply most days that I didn't want to go. On the rare day I would try to walk, I had to concentrate on every step and where and how I placed my feet. One day Russi came to tell me he'd been to the cardiac gym to ask Fiona (exercise physiologist in charge) why I wouldn't exercise or co-operate. Fiona told Russi that there must be something wrong if I wouldn't do anything. At last I had Norm and Fiona believing in me. At this stage the doctors also couldn't understand why I wouldn't do anything (the opposite to when I had my VAD). They ordered many tests and bloods to be taken. One day Russi came with a Birds Machine (improves the intake of air into the lungs by breathing deeper by providing short term mechanical ventilation), and left instructions about how to use it and for me to begin using it that night. A couple of hours later Russi called to tell me definitely DO NOT use the birds machine that night. The next morning Russi told me, a pathologist had called him with some results and advised him not to push me very hard. When the doctors did their rounds that morning I was told I had a lung embolism (obstruction of an artery, typically by a clot of blood or an air bubble.)

Mystery solved! From that moment everyone involved in my care did a 180 degree turn around in their attitude toward my care!

After the embolism was treated with Warfarin, my physical strength began improving. I began to communicate by using a few Makaton signs. I could sit out of bed in an armchair and was able to walk with a frame and then walking a little further. Russi still had a wheelchair ready just in case I needed it. Over time Russi and I became good friends. He brought in photos of his trip to Namibia and of his children. The nurses now wanted me to dress in day clothes for so-called psychological well-being. How can you pretend you're at home when in a hospital room clearly unwell surrounded by nurses and can hardly move? It didn't happen.

After being assessed by an Occupational Therapist (OT) I began doing writing exercises in pre-school activity books, learning to write again. Food wasn't such a problem now as I had a slight appetite and enjoyed the vegetarian and vegan food so much more than meat. My breathing was easier, I could actually get the balls in a small breathing apparatus. This was to improve my breathing and inflate my lungs.

The tablets didn't leave me feeling as sick and with a vile aftertaste as before. As the anti-rejection medication was tweaked to suit me, my sleeping improved with a regular nightly sleeping tablet. I could now have a shower and have my hair washed, with a couple of nurs-

es helping. It was absolutely wonderful to feel clean.

I was still frustrated by the fact that I couldn't talk or walk very much by myself. I couldn't pull a tissue from a tissue box nor flush the toilet. I wondered if they were ever able to fix my body.

My progression slowly headed in the right direction but being healthy again was still thwarted several times in the coming weeks. Two or three weeks after I was strong enough to sit up and actually walk unsteadily, my lungs filled with fluid. I required bilateral pleural drainage. My chest was pierced on my right side by a trainee surgeon and drained into a jar on the floor overnight. The next afternoon my left side was drained. Both sides were drained separately in case my lung collapsed. One liter of fluid was drained from each lung. Out of all the procedures I had, this would have to be the most painful. A local anesthetic can only be inserted so far into the chest then a pair of clippers cut through the deeper tissue to the pleural cavity. This was done before a drain can be inserted and sutured to enable drainage. Norm had gone back to Quairading again to check his house. My sister Elaine stayed falling asleep by my side for the whole time I had these drains.

*A typical week seemed like one step forward and constantly two backwards. On **October 9** I had more blood tests and a CT scan at 7pm and was still on morphine. **October 10**, Russi managed to take me for a very short walk before I had another Octogram infusion. This was immunoglobulin containing a broad spectrum of anti-bodies against infectious agents. **October 11** I had two bags of platelets.*

*Monday **12th October** my hemoglobin was low which meant I needed heamdyalisis ....even Russi the physio wouldn't take me for a walk! The next day I had plasma pheresis again for maybe the 10th or 12th time. Somewhere in between all the other procedures I had two heart biopsies, that were done to check for rejection. These are* *very similar to an angiogram but instead a small piece of the heart muscle is snipped off for biopsy.*

This procedure like most of them isn't very pleasant either. The nurses, office staff, and visitors couldn't find me and often asked me where had I been and commented on how busy I was. It seemed like the never-ending story.

A few days after the embolism, I decided I was going home. I woke up early, organized my room, showered, got dressed in day clothes, packed up my things and happily waited for the cardiac team. As soon as they saw me they asked me what I thought I was doing? I cheerfully told them 'I am going home today."

They sternly told me I wasn't going anywhere... after they'd finished laughing. After this I decided to co-operate and do whatever they told me. Even when someone rocked up with a wheelchair to take me somewhere, I gave up asking why, where or what. I'd had enough tests and procedures to last me a lifetime. They could have taken me anywhere I wouldn't have known the difference.

Another time I was to have IV Phenergan (promethazine)... after the first half hour I thrashed around the bed holding my head as I had the worst headache ever imagined. Thankfully my bed rails were always up as I was still a falls risk. The cardiac registrar Si-an had to stay with me for the rest of the day in case my intolerance became life threatening.

As my rejection was still high I was given Rituximab (an IV man - made antibody drug) also sometimes used for chemotherapy. It is light sensitive and has to be covered in black plastic and has to be handled carefully with purple gloves and disposed of in special bags. After this I looked like a sunburnt pixie and I had diarrhea!

It wasn't all bad, one night when I was extremely restless I told a nurse I couldn't sleep on the air mattress anymore and she organized an ordinary mattress, although I craved the comfort of my own bed. The difference was instant and wonderful relief.

I think it was the same day I was transferred to another room away from the nurse's desk. A support worker brought Teoni in to see me which was amazing. I was so glad to see her and she was thrilled to see me. . She brought me a teddy bear as a Christmas present. My nephew sent me a Scottish doll dressed in a Scottish soldier's uniform. He said it was to guard me. At this stage I could not remember how long I had been in hospital but at least I was now allowed out of the ward for the first time; downstairs to the coffee shop in a wheelchair with Norm if I had a nurse escort. Simon, a senior nurse volunteered. Having the wind in my face and being outside was wonderful.

I saw Michelle, a former nurse who had previously been my special nurse who looked after me when transferred from ICU after Fremantle Hospital. She couldn't believe how well I looked nor what I'd been through. From then on, back in the ward, my bed was moved from room to room for some unknown reason, until finally they put me over the other side from CCU to Ward 4, the regular non acute cardiac ward. This was a good sign I had improved significantly enough and would soon be going home. By this stage with my own pillow and doona and a few homely comforts, CCU and ward 4 were like home away from home.

As I regained my strength and motivation my sister Elaine bought *some ¾ shorts from the op shop for me to wear as day clothes and to the gym. My weight was regularly changing. Each night she'd take my washing and bring back clean clothes. By now I was attending the gym and walking reasonably well on the treadmill and doing weights. Since the last time I'd been at the gym, with my VAD before my transplant, I'd lost 9 kilos. When I first started exercising post-transplant my strength was almost nil. From my wheelchair, I'd go through the motions of each exercise with my hands made into a fist without any weights. Although my gym routine appeared simple and easy, it didn't take very long before I was much fitter and stronger.*

Some of the nurses still thought I was being lazy as they never saw me walking around the ward. Julie, one of the cardiac team nurses, told me it was all about being seen. From then on I made sure I walked when all the nurses were having changeover, and when they were all around I'd make myself clearly visible and would often speak to all of them.

A few of the nurses I now knew rather well told me I was really funny in the beginning, trying to exercise, my arms and head would flop everywhere and I looked like a rag doll. They were pleased to hear me trying to speak in short sentences, as before they couldn't understand anything I said. I thought I was making sense. A nurse from Ireland asked if I had any words of wisdom I'd learned from my experience.

I told her that being humble was something I intended to follow from now on and if you want to do anything, don't wait, just do it!

She told me this was the deciding factor for her to return home to Ireland to live.

After a while I was becoming irritable and tired again and just wanted to go home. The doctors began to make arrangements for me to be discharged. They had decided I still required some anti-rejection therapy and discussed me having Total Lymphatic Irradiation (TLI) as an outpatient after I regained some of my strength. They organized another person who'd had TLI eight years previously to come in to see me, as proof it works and explain the procedure. If there was a positive having TLI, it was that no more heart biopsies were required. The TLI renders the biopsies inaccurate. My legs still looked like keg barrels and I had to wear soft socks to protect my sore feet. Even at this stage I kept trying to talk but couldn't make myself heard very often.

Before discharge, Norm bought me some clothes to wear home which consisted of my best trousers, no knickers, a few old t-shirts and two pajama tops. I also had an ear, nose and throat (ENT) specialist visit in case my trachea had been damaged. He sprayed the back of my throat with a local anesthetic before asking me to swallow a tube with a light on the end so he could look at my throat. As my throat was clear he suggested I have speech therapy. I gagged for the rest of the day. Also, an Occupational Therapist (OT) had to visit my home to check if any modifications were necessary for me. I had a raised chair above the toilet, another in the shower and the hospital carpenters made a raised platform for an armchair for me to sit in.

CHAPTER 11

DISCHARGE & HOME

My enthusiasm to leave the security of hospital was extremely limited. I knew I had to leave and wanted to, but was very reluctant. The transition to home happened in stages. I was allowed some day leave (2 hours) so we went to Kings Park where I had a choc milk. It was fantastic to go somewhere again. This was followed by a day visit home. Then an overnight at home before actually being discharged altogether from hospital. After sleeping in the hospital beds, mine was pure luxury. I had many Do s and don'ts to follow over the next few weeks. Although I could walk, I still felt very weak and it was only small distances before becoming very breathless. My muscles still hurt... I had very little appetite, was tired, very little energy and the tablets still made me feel sick. I had read the heart muscle is the strongest in the body and thought mine must be strong as all the others felt very weak. I was still mostly in a wheel chair which Norm helped me with particularly when I was at the hospital.

I arrived home on day 43, whether this is inclusive of ICU I haven't the foggiest. I still had a long way to go. My house wasn't very tidy when I walked inside, I was very disappointed. I had refused agency home help as I'd had this when Teoni was born and on one hand it was sort of useful on the other, more of a nuisance. It tied me down too much. My sister Elaine was already back home in Gunnedah NSW, which left Norm and Jamie together at my house. Norm said he didn't care and Jamie said I was too fussy. The next day I commenced to clean up as best I could. For the first time since my transplant I became rather disillusioned about what had happened. Guilty that I had someone else's heart beating inside me, the fragility of life and the uncertainty of the future. I felt I was on an emotional roller coaster and didn't like my life anymore.

My first dinner at home... I felt like potato salad and it was delicious. My tastes had definitely changed. The most significant and long lasting has been: before transplant I'd drink 5-6 cups of coffee daily. The moment my eyes opened in CCU, tea was and has been my favorite hot drink since. My friends and family are rather amused by the switch from coffee to tea. I rarely drink coffee anymore. Both Norm and Jamie made a huge effort to cook and do lots of different things to help me, except clean. The second night I was home, day 45, for the first time I slept ALL night. A few good uninterrupted night sleeps later, I felt so much better than I had and began to brighten up.

For the next few weeks I/we had to avoid places where it might be possible to pick up an infection. We were told when we had hospital appointments to walk right around another way to stay away from ICU. I had to stay at home as much as possible.

I wasn't allowed to do any gardening or touch soil. Be as clean as possible: wiping benches down daily, changing dish clothes daily, only eating fresh in date washed food and cold food had to be cold and hot food had to be hot. I had to use one board for cutting vegetables and another for meat. I wasn't allowed to have deli food, as it could be reheated, for quick sale. And definitely no leftover foods.

Margot Maurice

There are a few guidelines regarding food that is best followed post-transplant especially in the early days. There's a post-transplant list of what is and isn't allowed. I still adhere to a few of these do's and don'ts but now have relaxed most of them within reason.

I was quickly introduced to the post-transplant follow up regime which commenced a week after discharge. I was given handouts for this, to make things easier. The gym routine had to be adhered to reasonably strictly three times per week. I could now do a slow five minutes on the bike. The other gym members were a huge resource and support especially for the first six months or so until I managed to build up some stamina. They all knew what I'd been through and were exceptionally supportive. I measured my improvement by how high I could lift my arms, how many balls I could blow on the thingamajig blower to inflate my lungs, enabling me to breathe deeper.

I stayed at the RPH gym for six years and loved every minute.

No-one ever pushed me to do more, only encouraged me to do what I could, which left me extremely grateful not to have any added pressure in my life. Weekly speech therapy sessions as an outpatient were on the agenda for a few weeks until the funding ran out. It is difficult to say if these sessions helped or not.

Week 9... I began with total lymphoid irradiation (TLI) for the treatment of early or recurrent heart transplant rejection.

TLI daily for 4-5 days or that's my recollection. I had an initial radiation clinic visit where the procedure was explained. I was measured and a small dot tattooed where the radiation would be targeted. The radiation room was tucked away beneath the hospital; it was freezing cold and the metal table was cold and bare. I had a wafer thin anti-nausea tablet half an hour before each radiation visit. After the 3rd day I was feeling more tired than ever and again not feeling like myself. I saw the TLI doctor once prior to TLI, then numerous post follow up blood tests and doctor check-ups at regular intervals later. I wasn't allowed to go to the gym, had to reduce my prednisolone dosage. That is a steroid. It prevents the release of substances in the body that cause inflammation and stop the mycophenolate completely.

Mycophenolate (CellCept) is used with other medications to help prevent transplant organ rejection or an attack of the transplanted organ by the immune system of the person receiving the organ.

Also in people who have received kidney, heart, and liver transplants.

After every hospital visit we'd always have a coffee. There were always a few people having coffee we knew and these visit/appointments became regular social occasions. It was a difficult and joyful time mixed together.

For a very long time I had to be in a wheelchair when I went out. I needed a walking stick to walk anywhere even around my house. I still needed a lot of rest as I was still breathless on exertion. I remember my first grocery shopping trip. After walking one aisle I felt as though I'd walked 100 kilometers s and couldn't go any further. Teoni was only allowed to have regular short visits home. I found it very difficult dealing with my own changed needs, combined with Teoni's needs as it compounded my situation significantly. Although she loved being with Owen, it must have been a confusing time for her. Sadly, her skill level had definitely regressed. It has taken a long time to resume and for her to gain a former version of skills she'd had previously.

Gradually the walking stick wasn't required as my walking became stronger. Teoni graduated from visiting to the odd overnight stay as

Margot Maurice

I grew stronger. These overnight stays increased to two nights, then three nights and so on. It was 15 months - two years post-op before she came home permanently.

Even now she stays one night/or sometimes a week at Owens.

Spiritually, this experience made me realize I am not very spiritual as I had previously thought, although I do attend church and communion sometimes. Emotionally, I think I was just too sick to care and because of the support, pulled through without a lot of drama and am forever grateful for my recovery and everyone involved in my care. Church and prayer is still a haven for Norm and since helping me, he attends the monthly Healing Service held the first Tuesday of every month.

It was and still is, very difficult to draw blood from me. Some phlebotomists use heat, rubbing or whatever they think might work but not many are able to draw my blood the first go, or second or third. I've had phlebitis, severe bruising, collapsed veins, and every other blood related trauma from blood tests or IV infusions. Only once have I been in tears when a guy at RPH tried four-five times and hurt like crazy. It was after this I found out they can only try twice, I think. Usually it is taken from the back of the hand or above my elbow. Once I went to two clinics where, neither could take my blood. They finally advised me to go to either a hospital clinic or a clinic that has at least two phlebotomists. Now it doesn't matter what procedure or test I have. I have a strong aversion to all medical procedures and tests of any nature.

I know I am ever so appreciative of having a nursing background. With any medical terminology, explanation, procedures, and tests it has helped tremendously. I understood the basics of why, what, where and how of the anatomy, physiology of the body plus procedures and tests. In the end I never asked where I was going or why. I just hopped in the wheelchair and did whatever I was told to do. I learned the best way to handle procedures was to hold my breath or freeze (grin and bear it attitude); it didn't matter how much it hurt, it hurt a whole lot less and was quicker if I went with the flow, co-operated and clenched my teeth. The following April, Allen another heart recipient and I attended a Q and A function for an education/information group of approximately 200 nurses, to answer any queries or questions they had about transplants and CADS. Because Allen and I were totally different ends of the recovery spectrum it was a really good opportunity for me to give my point of view about ICU and various nursing practices during my hospital admissions.

After the initial bombardment of appointments, tests and procedures we settled down into a muddled routine but still a routine that we became used to and knew what to expect. Now it is all rather routine: I have six monthly AHFCTS clinic visits. These consist routinely of a fasting blood test, an ECG and chest x-ray prior to clinic. At clinic we are seen by either a cardiologist, the registrar or Clare the Clinical Nurse Specialist, depending on how much help we need and what is required. Every year or two (I think) a Debutamine echo is required. A **Dobutamine** Stress **Echo** (DSE) is a specialized ultrasound examination where a medication, **(Dobutamine)** is used to replicate the effect of exercise by increasing the heart rate. This test is recommended for patients who, for many different reasons, cannot walk on a treadmill.

An IV is inserted and while an echo is being performed you're given Debutamine to speed up the heart to beat faster and faster at a pre-determined level. My heart is extremely difficult to slow down after. I need some IV medication to reverse the procedure. Not very pleasant. I'm always relieved when it's finished.

Margot Maurice

Yearly dental checkups, a flu vaccination, two yearly pap smear, regular exercise preferably in a gym, we need to keep an eye on weight and if it goes up a kilogram in 24 hours call the clinic.

(1kilogram is a 1 liter of fluid), this can be a sign not only of fluid retention but also of rejection. Transplant recipients aren't allowed live vaccines or anti-inflammatories. My regular GP does a six monthly health management plan which entitles the patient to so many subsidized ancillary sessions. A yearly skin checkup is strongly advised. The anti-rejection medications increase the possibility of skin cancer by 200%. My skin doctor wants me to come in for a full body check every 4 months. He says skin cancer needs to be detected early and tells me, after a transplant if all the things you have had to contend with don't kill you, then skin cancer will. He also has me on Vitamin A five days a week, Vitamin B 5 daily (we need to stay out of the sun), Nicotinamide daily and daily Magnesium tablets.

Every year on 9/11, I go to St Georges Cathedral in town to say prayers and light a candle in memory of my donor. I am trying to look after and honor my transplant heart. I go to the gym for a few months then slacken off then begin again. At the moment I go to the gym at Curtin University and I am in the process of changing to a regular gym, closer to home with more regular opening hours. Teoni and I do the four kilometer, City to Surf walk each year. It is not much, but it is all I am capable of doing. It took 2 years to write a letter to my donor's family and to genuinely say thank you. I definitely felt much more alive when I had my VAD (long term use is an unknown). Having a transplant does enable more freedom. It was approximately 2-3 years after my transplant to gradually regain my strength and feel any normality again in my life. Since then I am grateful to feel okay, though still not one hundred per cent right.

A visual journey of my illness was documented by Norm. He would often take pictures or video a scene. Often we'd arrange and rearrange everything in a room or outside for him to set up and capture what was happening. These homemade DVDs took hours of work for him. He was always easy to find well into the night and the early hours of each morning editing chunks of video footage, dubbing on overlays of sound and finding special effects to produce some really interesting and great homemade memories.

Eventually I was stronger. Teoni had returned home and it was getting closer for Norm to go home to Quairading. We'd taken him to high-tea as a thank you for helping out. Every weekend for a month or so we'd travel the 200 plus kilometers to clean, tidy and organize his house for him to move back. The last weekend we'd brought groceries to take to Quairading. Then we came back to Perth for him to finally pack up his clothes before returning home.

The day before he was to leave, he woke me up about six o'clock in the morning, wanting me to take him to hospital NOW! He was clutching his chest and was beside himself with chest pain. That drive was one of the scariest I'd ever done. I kept telling him to breathe properly and if he died on me in my car I wasn't talking to him ever again. His troponin was raised which meant he'd had a slight heart attack. A troponin test measures the levels of troponin T or troponin I proteins in the blood. These proteins are released when the heart muscle has been damaged, such as occurs with a heart attack. The more damage there is to the heart, the greater the amount of troponin T and I there will be in the blood.

He stayed in Fremantle hospital for a few days, had an angiogram, further heart tests and wasn't allowed to return to Quairading in the near future!

Thankfully Teoni had stayed asleep as it was always problematic with her in an emergency situation. Now the carer became the cared for- our roles had reversed. Norm has only ever been back to his home in Quairading for a few days here and there. Norm is still in Perth 8.5 years down the track. He stayed at my house for another year before relocating to his son's house not far away. His son is offshore working in Mongolia and Norm is house sitting and looking after Fred, the dog!

I found it very difficult to walk when the time came for my post-transplant checks as my legs often swelled. Over time my left leg healed and hasn't been bothersome for some four years now. My right leg still becomes very swollen with fluid. The summer heat and walking longer distances exacerbates the soreness and difficulty I have. A special stocking relieves the fluid retention somewhat sometimes. If my leg felt better and I didn't occasionally become breathless, I'd feel fantastic. Often I have the odd time when I'm not feeling well or need to walk a long way and do use the ACROD, Disability Parking permit then someone inevitably questions me about taking a disability bay. Although I am very much in favor of others keeping an eye out like this, it adds to me feeling self-consciousness about the whole deal.

A Postscript from Rhonda regarding her two children:

Since my transplant Jamie bleary eyed told me he actually said goodbye to me while I was in ICU. The doctors had told everyone my chances of surviving would be a miracle.

I explained to Teoni, "Mummy was very sick and am better now I have a 'new' heart."

She seems to understand this concept and used to ask "how's your new heart going?" but now often asks if I am okay?"

CHAPTER 12

Some thoughts from the author.

During procedures such as many Rhonda had endured, she was being given morphine or other similar drugs of the hallucinogen group. These drugs cause many people to see or sense things that are not real. You would have read about the problems the previous two Transplant patients also had with these drugs.

Last year I was given morphine in spite of having information listed with the medical staff in two different hospitals as to what I either had allergic reactions to or stated I did not want to be given. Two of the main offending drugs for me are morphine and codeine yet both were administered to me when I was unconscious with disastrous results. I don't know what one can do if our wishes are not adhered to other than lodge some complaint. I understand it makes the patient easier to manage if drugged but this is not necessarily in the best interest of the patient.

These drugs seem to have adverse effects on many people who have been prescribed them, yet seem to still be administered to most patients in most hospitals. Easier for the nurses but certainly not for patients.

……………………………………………………..

Margot Maurice

These stories are true and are, as submitted to me for this book. It exemplifies the strength of the human spirit in all three stories yet are still quite different. One never knows how they would cope until put into a similar situation.

The length of recovery of each one has been very different; different side issues, different coping mechanisms, but above all I am eternally grateful to all three for allowing me to use their amazing stories. As Rhonda has succinctly said, "It is unbelievable what we get through and by the grace of our God, we cope."

CHAPTER 13

A word of advice

Early days of my cardiomyopathy in 1984 I often had bouts of sadness at not qualifying for a heart transplant as that appeared to be my only option of staying alive. I had no idea what this entailed of course. However since reading and editing the transplant stories of these three members of Cardiomyopathy Australia, I am now thankful I was able to not need to have a transplant and thank all my general practitioners and medical specialists over the last thirty three years that have been involved in my case and continue to give me good advice and are keeping me alive.

I have been told more than once that the medicos are learning a lot from my longevity and several have now accepted that science does not always have all the answers.

I have had several of the procedures that the three transplant stories have reported, the difference being that I have been fortunate enough over these years to survive and avoid over the years the need to be placed on a transplant list mainly because I have either been too old, or with little chance of survival and I am grateful for their advice. It is good to be confident that one's doctors have the interest of the patient at heart and not just the interest of research which is sometimes at the ultimate cost of a patient. I know doctors don't want to lose a patient but the excitement of the outcome of research is sometimes an ego trip when something new is discovered through research.

Presently my specialists are not keen to upset the status quo and they often remark that my positive attitude appears to help me stay on the periphery of this life threatening condition.

I have my goals and my only long term one is, I would like to be around to celebrate my 90th birthday. This goal is made up of regular daily goals to be around for the next day. If I continue to stick to these goals I will very possibly make my long term one as taking these small bites of daily goals will automatically result in my long term one. I have stated though that I reserve the right to change my mind about this at any time in the future.

I have been told by my cardiologist that no one really knows when one has reached the end of their human life but determination goes a long way to achieving my ultimate. This will require constant regular meditation and affirmations; two things I have done for most of my life so it will be more of the same. But there is always fate and in my case it hasn't been in my agenda to need a transplant. I am lucky.

I have no fear of dying as when the time comes for me to leave this mortal coil, I will be ready for my next adventure. I am now in my 85th year so I can't complain. I spend most of my days writing and looking after myself with the help of my wonderful partner, John Gallagher.

I do believe in everlasting life but not in my present form. We change our form according to where we are; similar to being spiritually suitably dressed for any occasion.

When in Rome do as the Romans do.

I hope you have found this book about heart transplants interesting. We sometimes tend to think there is one size that fits all in many things in life but organ transplant in this book really shows how different we all are.

I have found it interesting and I hope that you, the reader, will not dismiss some of the theories that may be a little 'way out' to you. Remember everything is possible.

FINAL WORDS AND ACKNOWLEDGMENTS

"I bless my late parents as well as my late maternal grandmother for breeding into me a strong, intuitive and positive mind and for teaching me that 'if it is to be, it's up to me.'

"I trust that readers will be able to learn something from the stories in this book and realize we are all very different and therefore handle our health and illness in a variety of ways.

I attribute my survival from cardiomyopathy since the 1984 prognosis to many factors: Developments in medication and diagnostic techniques, the love from my partner and fellow author John J. Gallagher as well as my daughter Vanda Leigh and granddaughter Mondanna Leigh.

I encourage those with a severe health problem to understand there is more of the doctor in your God than perhaps God in your doctor.

Don't let any prognosis define the length of your life. Live every day as you choose and fill it with laughter and fun then each night before you go to sleep, give thanks to 'your God' for yet another day."

Special thanks to Ryan Ashcroft (www.loveyourcovers.com) for his work on the cover art; and to Yvonne Betancourt (www.ebook-format.com) for her work on the interior design.

Blessings
Margot Maurice.

OTHER BOOKS BY THIS AUTHOR

'Six Months to Live... my cardiomyopathy story of Mind over Medicine.'

Kindle Ebook & Paper book.

'The Eleventh Hour... sequel to Six Months to Live.' Kindle Ebook & Paper book.

'Cardiomyopathy...Keeping you on Track.' Celebratory book for 20th Anniversary of Cardiomyopathy Australia. Kindle Ebook.

'The Seven Recurring Questions of Life.' Co-written with John J. Gallagher. Kindle Ebook.

All books available on Amazon books, Goodreads & other online booksellers.

For more information, please visit my website at:

www.gallagherandmauricebooks.com

www.ingramcontent.com/pod-product-compliance
Lightning Source LLC
Chambersburg PA
CBHW070105210526
45170CB00013B/755